PHARMACY LAW SIMPLIFIED

NORTH CAROLINA MPJE® STUDY GUIDE

2014 EDITION

BY
DAVID A HECKMAN, PHARMD

The author does not assume and hereby disclaims any liability to any party for losses, damages, and/or failures caused by error or omission, regardless of whether such error or omission resulted from negligence, oversight, accident, or any other cause.

This publication is not a substitute for legal advice. For legal advice, consult a legal professional.

This publication does not contain actual exam content.

MPJE®, NAPLEX®, and NABP® are federally registered trademarks of the National Association of Boards of Pharmacy (NABP®). The National Association of Boards of Pharmacy (NABP®) does not endorse, authorize, or sponsor this, or any other, study guide.

Book cover designed by **Keeling Design & Media, Inc.**

Published by Heckman Media
First edition published 2013 © David A. Heckman

Printed in the United States of America

INTRODUCTION

This book was created for individuals preparing for pharmacist licensure in North Carolina. To save you time and to facilitate easy understanding and quick learning, laws and rules have been simplified into a question-and-answer format. Now you can focus on what is important - studying key points and passing the exam.

- Computer-based exam.
- $210 enrollment fee.
- Administered at Pearson VUE Testing Centers.
- 90 multiple choice questions.
- 120 minutes to complete exam.
- Scoring is scaled from 0-100.
- Earn a scaled score of 75 or higher to pass.

NORTH CAROLINA
PHARMACY LAWS AND RULES
SIMPLIFIED

What are common abbreviations for the "North Carolina Board of Pharmacy?"
- The Board.
- NCBOP.

Why was the NCBOP created?
To enforce the North Carolina Pharmacy Practice Act and other laws concerning the distribution and use of drugs.

How does the NCBOP enforce pharmacy laws?
Through the adoption and application of reasonable rules (the "North Carolina Pharmacy Rules," which are available on the NCBOP website).

Does the NCBOP support substance abuse rehabilitation for pharmacists?
Yes, by funding the North Carolina Pharmacist Recovery Network (NCPRN), a program for pharmacists addicted to controlled substances and/or alcohol.

How is the NCPRN funded?
From fees (e.g. pharmacist licensing fees).

How many Board members comprise the NCBOP?
6 members.

How are the 6 Board members chosen?
- 5 are NC licensed pharmacists elected by other NC pharmacists.
- 1 is an NC resident appointed by the NC Governor to represent the public.

Are you required to live in NC to serve on the Board?
Yes, all candidates must reside in NC at the time of their election/appointment and throughout their term of service.

Does the Governor have to choose a pharmacist?
No, in fact the Board member appointed by the Governor cannot be a healthcare professional or a healthcare student, and he/she cannot be married to a healthcare professional or healthcare student.

Who participates in the election of NCBOP members?
Every pharmacist that is licensed and residing in NC.

Where do Board member candidates come from?
Each of the five pharmacist-elected Board members represents one of five geographic locations in North Carolina.

Who can nominate a candidate for Board election?
- The Committee on Nominations.
- Ten eligible voters from one of the five geographic areas.

When do nominations close?
March 15TH.

When is the Board of Pharmacy Election held?
Every May when there is a vacant Board member seat.

How do you cast your ballot for a Board election?
Electronically, but paper ballots are available upon request.

When are ballots due?
Ballots must be submitted or postmarked (for paper ballots) by May 15TH.

How long is one term for a Board member?
5 years.

What are the Board member term limits?
Board members can serve up to two consecutive five year terms.

Note: after serving two consecutive terms, a member can serve again after sitting out at least one term.

If chosen to serve on the Board, what must that new member do next?
Appear at their county courthouse within 10 days to take an oath.

How much do Board members get paid?
Up to $100/day on days they conduct "official business of the Board."

Does the Board have a President and Vice President?
Yes, the Board elects its own president and vice president from among the members.

For the Board to make official decisions, how many members must be present?
4 members.

What is the minimum number of times the Board must convene each year?
At least twice annually to administer tests (i.e. NAPLEX® and MPJE®).
Note: these exams are administered much more frequently now by computer at testing centers across the country.

How does the Board keep track of pharmacists and pharmacy owners?
They maintain a list of licensees and permit holders.

Who does the Board report to?
The Board reports to the Governor and the head of each house of the General Assembly

Does the NCBOP have any full-time employees?
Yes, the Board employs an Executive Director to work full-time as the
Secretary/Treasurer (to perform administrative tasks) and other personnel.

Do employees of the Board only make up to $100/day like the Board members?
No, compensation for Board employees is different and is determined by the
Board.

Who grants approval for purchases made by the Board?
The Governor and the Council of the State approve the Board for
rentals/purchases.

Does the Executive Director of the Board have any law enforcement authority?
Yes, if the NC Pharmacy Practice Act is violated, the Executive Director of the
Board has the authority to conduct an investigation and prosecute the violator in a
Board hearing.

Does the Board have the right to access pharmacy prescription files?
Yes.

Can the NC Pharmacy Act ever be waived?
Yes, if a state of emergency or disaster is declared then the NCBOP can waive the
act to allow drugs, devices, and professional services to be provided to the public.

What types of events must be reported to the NCBOP and in what time frame?
Disasters, accidents, thefts, or emergencies that could affect the purity, strength,
and/or labeling of drugs or devices must be reported to the NCBOP within 10
days.

In what ways can a technician be punished by the Board?
- Letters of reprimand.
- Registration suspensions.
- Registration revocations.
- Registration denials.

If you lie on an application for a pharmacist license or pharmacy permit, can you be punished by the Board?
Yes.

As a licensed pharmacist, if you plead nolo contendere (no contest) to a felony involving drugs, can the Board punish you?
Yes.

If you abuse drugs and are unfit to work as a result, can the Board punish you?
Yes.

If you willfully violate the laws/rules of the Board, can the Board punish you?
Yes.

If you develop a physical or mental disability, can the Board place limitations or restrictions on your license?
Yes.

If a pharmacist refills a 30-day supply of medication upon request from a patient every 7 days, is this okay.
No, this could be considered negligence since it is obvious that the patient may be taking more than the prescribed amount.

How exactly can the NCBOP punish a pharmacist?
- Letters of reprimand.
- Registration suspensions.
- License restrictions.
- License suspensions.
- License revocations.
- License denials.

What prompts the Board to punish a licensee or permit holder?
- Lied or omitted information to get licensee or permit.
  - o Licenses and permits acquired by deception are considered void.
- Found guilty of or pled nolo contendere (no contest) to a felony involving pharmacy and/or drugs.
- Used drugs to extent that one is unfit to practice pharmacy.
- Used deception in the practice of pharmacy which led to harming, potentially harming, and/or defrauding the public.
  - o e.g. telling a customer that they should purchase cough syrup even though they are coughing up blood just so you can make money off of the sale of the cough syrup.
- Failed to comply with pharmacy laws.
- Practiced or helped someone practice pharmacy without a license.
- Practiced pharmacy with negligence.

What are possible NCBOP disciplinary actions?
- Letter of reprimand.
- Suspension of license.
- Restriction of license.
- Revocation of license.
- Refusal to grant or renew a license.
- Requirement fro remedial education.

True or False. If a pharmacist does not pay child support fees, his or her license can be revoked?
True, the license can be reinstated once the clerk of the superior court certifies that the child support fees have been paid.

If the NCBOP tries to limit a pharmacist's rights, duties, and/or privileges, what is that pharmacist entitled to?
A hearing.

Is a hearing the only option?
No, the dispute may be settled informally.

What can be done if a pharmacist believes the NCBOP has acted in a way that affects his or her rights, duties, or privileges?
The pharmacist can file a request for a hearing.
Note: such a request may be denied by the Board.

The NCBOP must notify you of the details (e.g. meeting time) of the hearing at least how many days before the hearing?
15 days.

What is a contested hearing?
A hearing in which there are two parties that disagree.

Who shall hear a contested case?
Hearings shall be conducted by the Board, a panel of a majority of Board members, or an administrative law judge.

When should a Board member disqualify him or herself from hearing a contested case?
When he or she is unable to perform all duties impartially.

What should be done if one of the parties in a contested case believes one of the Board members is personally biased?
A petition for disqualification of the member should be filed.

If three or more members of the Board are disqualified by such a petition, then who shall hear the contested case?
An administrative law judge.

Decisions for all cases heard by the Board will be issued within how many days?
Within 60 days after the next regularly scheduled Board meeting following the close of the hearing.
What is the case is heard by an administrative law judge?
Then the decision will be rendered within 45 days.

If a non-pharmacist owns a pharmacy, can he/she obtain a pharmacy permit before securing management/staff?
No, the owner must be able to name the pharmacist-manager and all other pharmacy personnel in the pharmacy permit application.

Do employee changes have to be reported?
Yes, the pharmacist-manager must notify the NCBOP within 30 days of significant changes in pharmacy personnel.

You work for a free clinic with a mobile pharmacy. Since the pharmacy moves from one location to another, how many permits must it hold?
Only one pharmacy permit is required, but each location from which drugs are dispensed must be reported to the NCBOP.

Doctors call you to ask if they must register with the NCBOP to dispense drugs from their office. What do you tell them?
Prescribers that dispense drugs for a fee are required to register annually with the NCBOP.
Note: physician dispensing still has to comply with the same drug distribution laws that apply to pharmacists (e.g. packaging, labeling, and record-keeping laws).

What is the initial fee for a pharmacy permit?
$500.

What is the annual renewal fee for a pharmacy permit?
$200.

What is the late renewal fee for a pharmacy permit?
$400.

What is the fee to transfer ownership of a pharmacy?
$500.

If physically located out-of-state, does a pharmacy doing business in NC have to hold a NC pharmacy permit?
Yes and the permit must be renewed annually.

What if the out-of-state pharmacy does business by mail?
Even if prescription drugs are dispensed from out of state via mail (or by any other means), the dispensing pharmacy is still required to get a permit from the NCBOP.

You apply for a pharmacy permit from out-of-state. Can your application be affected by your record with another state's board of pharmacy?
Yes, if you have been formally disciplined for something pharmacy-related in another state, the NCBOP can deny your application for a permit.

Can an internet pharmacy obtain a permit from the NCBOP?
Yes, but only if the pharmacy is certified by the NABP® as a Verified Internet Pharmacy Practice Site (VIPPS).

If your pharmacy changes owners, do you have to obtain a new pharmacy permit?
Yes.

Before the Board will issue the original pharmacy permit (this does not apply to renewals), who must personally appear before the Board?
The proposed pharmacist-manager and the person in charge of the business (e.g. the owner) must appear before the Board.

Pharmacies that dispense drugs from out-of-state must provide _____ to its customers?
A toll-free phone number on the prescription label where a pharmacist at the facility can be contacted.

When does the aforementioned phone service have to be made available to customers?
During the pharmacy's normal business hours, a minimum of 6 days/week and 40 hours/week.

If it appears that a drug dispensed by an out-of-state pharmacy contributed to the death of a customer, in what time frame must that pharmacy notify the NCBOP?
Once the pharmacy is aware, they have 14 days to report it.

If an out-of-state pharmacy is disciplined by any Board of Pharmacy, in what time frame must they notify the NCBOP?
5 days.

If an out-of-state pharmacy is disciplined by its own state board, is it likely to be disciplined by the NCBOP?
Yes.

If you dispense medical oxygen, how much oxygen must be dispensed as a backup supply?
The equivalent of 24 hours of therapy and supplies must be dispensed as backup supply.

I know that I must notify the Board if there is a change in pharmacist-managers, but does the Board collect a fee?
Yes, the fee to change a pharmacist-manager is $35.

If your pharmacy wants to sell medical devices, will you need a separate permit?
No, businesses holding a pharmacy permit do not need a separate device permit to sell medical devices.

If you hold a pharmacy permit, do you need a separate medical equipment permit to sell medical equipment?
No, as with the device permit, a medical equipment permit is not needed for businesses that already hold a pharmacy permit.

What is the fee for making changes in pharmacy personnel?
$35.

Which pharmacy schools are approved by the NCBOP?
Schools accredited by the Accreditation Council for Pharmacy Education (ACPE).

What is the Board's expectation of pharmacy school graduates?
New graduates are expected to practice pharmacy safely.

True or false. A pharmacist license applicant can be subjected to a background check and fingerprinting.
True, the Department of Justice (DOJ) may run a background check on applicants and fingerprints may be required.

Which NC state regulatory body requires licensing of pharmacists?
The General Assembly of North Carolina.

What is the rationale for requiring licensure?
The standards that must be met to obtain licensure are intended help protect the citizens of North Carolina from the danger of placing a population in the hands of under-qualified pharmacists.

What exams must one pass to become a licensed pharmacist?
1. The North American Pharmacist Licensure Examination (NAPLEX®).
2. Multistate Pharmacy Jurisprudence Examination (MPJE®).

What score must you achieve on these exams to pass?
A scaled score of 75 or higher on both exams is required.

What is the purpose of pharmacist licensing exams?
To determine whether or not the applicant is capable of practicing pharmacy safely and properly.

How soon before the licensing exams must you submit the "Application for License by Examination" to the NCBOP?
At least 45 days before the exams.

Are applicants required to submit to a background check?
Yes.

Is proof of age required when applying for a license?
Yes (e.g. submit copy of birth certificate).

How much practical experience is required for licensure?
1500 hours.

Can practical experience be obtained out-of-state?
Yes, if the NCBOP approves the out-of-state experience.

When can a student begin logging the 1500 hours?
After completing two years of undergraduate coursework.

When does a pharmacist's license expire?
Every year on December 31ST.
Note: there is a 60 day grace period for license renewals.

Is it illegal to practice pharmacy with an expired license 30 days after the expiration date of December 31ST?
No, as mentioned above there is a grace period of 60 days.

If your personal mailing address or place of employment changes, how long do you have to notify the Board?
30 days.

If your place of employment changes, how long do you have to notify the Board?
30 days.

You are currently licensed in another state, but want to become licensed in NC. How do you get a NC license?
Reciprocate your current license to NC.

Can you reciprocate a license that was obtained through reciprocation?
No, you can only reciprocate a license obtained by examination.

How do you reciprocate your license to NC?
Fill out an application for reciprocation, pay the associated fee, and then pass the North Carolina MPJE®.

What documentation from the NCBOP must be visibly displayed in the pharmacy?
The pharmacist-manager's license, the pharmacy permit, and current renewals must be posted and visible to the public.
Note: each day that a license, permit, or renewal is not displayed is considered to be a separate punishable offense.

Are other pharmacists required to display their licenses in the pharmacy?
No, but all working pharmacists must have their licenses and most recent renewals available for inspection by the Board.

What is the fee for an "Application for License by Examination"?
$200.

What is the annual pharmacist license renewal fee?
$135.

Can a member of the US military get an extension to pay license or permit renewal fees at a later date?
Yes, provided they inform the Board before their license expires that they will need the extension.

If they fail to inform the NCBOP of their need for an extension before their license or permit expires, then what?
As long as they can prove that they were eligible for an extension, they will still be able to renew their license or permit.

What is the fee for obtaining a pharmacist license by reciprocation?
$600.

Can you order a duplicate copy of your license, permit, or registration? And if so, what is the fee?
Yes, it is free for government entities and $25 for everyone else.

True or False. The NCBOP has to fulfill any citizen's request for the licensed status of an individual.
True.

On what form does a student register for practical pharmacy training?
Application for Registration in Pharmacy Training Program.

On what form does a student report practical pharmacy experience?
Practical Pharmacy Experience Affidavit.

On what form does one apply for a pharmacist license?
Application for Examination and Registered Pharmacist Certificate.

On what form does one renew a pharmacist license?
Pharmacist License Annual Renewal Notice.

On what form does one apply for a pharmacy permit?
Application for Registration and Permit to Conduct a Pharmacy.

To obtain a pharmacist license, what form must be submitted to the NCBOP that proves completion of education?
Certificate of Graduation from College or School of Pharmacy.

Is continuing education required to keep your license active?
Yes.

How many hours of Continuing Education (CE) credits must a pharmacist earn each year?
15 hours.

How many of these CE hours must be obtained through contact programs?
8 hours.

What is a contact program?
A CE session where you have an opportunity for live 2-way communication with the presenter.

Does online CE count toward the annual 8 hour contact program requirement?
Yes, provided the live 2-way communication standard is met.

If a pharmacist earns more than 15 hours of CE in one year, can he/she carry over the extra CE hours to the next year?
Yes, up to 5 hours of CE may be carried over and applied to the next year's CE requirement.

How long must one maintain records of completed CE?
3 years.

Why is it important to maintain records of completed CE?
The Board can require pharmacists to submit proof of CE completion (i.e. certificates of credit) in a random audit.

Who approves continuing education programs?
The Board.

True or false. A high school student can be employed as a pharmacy technician.
True, a pharmacist-manager can hire a technician with a high school diploma or its equivalent, or someone enrolled in a program to earn a high school diploma or its equivalent.

Upon hire, uncertified pharmacy technicians must be trained. What topics must be covered in training?
- Pharmacy terminology.
- Pharmacy calculations.
- Drug dispensing systems.
- Prescription label requirements.
- Pharmacy laws/rules.
- Recordkeeping requirements.
- Documentation.
- Appropriate handling and storage of medications.

Once hired, in what time frame must technicians complete the training?
180 days.

Are all uncertified technicians required to undergo training?
No, if the technician is already registered with the NCBOP, then training is optional.
Note: the pharmacist-manager decides whether or not to provide training in these cases.

Are pharmacy technicians required to register with the Board?
Yes, within 30 days of beginning employment.

Is there a registration fee for pharmacy technicians?
Yes, the technician must pay a $30 registration fee, and registration must be renewed annually.

What is the deadline for pharmacy technician registration renewal?
December 31ST.
Note: there is a 60 day grace period, so as long as the Board receives the renewal fee/application within 60 days of December 31ST, there will be no penalties.

What are the some points regarding pharmacy technician registration with the NCBOP?
- Registration expires on December 31ST of each year.
- Registration must be renewed annually.
- The grace period for renewal is 60 days.
- Training is not required for students of a community college pharmacy technician program.
- Volunteer technicians at a free clinic do not need to register with the Board, but they must complete training.

What is the maximum legal pharmacist-to-technician ratio?
One pharmacist to two technicians.
**Exception: with written approval from the Board, this ratio can be exceeded (more technicians), but any additional technicians must be <u>certified</u> technicians.

Let's say you have submitted a request for additional technicians, but 35 days have gone by and you have not heard from the Board. What do you do now?
Keep waiting, the NCBOP is required to respond to these requests within 60 days.
Note: if you receive disapproval, the Board must provide a reasonable explanation for the disapproval.

What activities are within the scope of pharmacy practice?
- Processing medication orders.
- Compounding drugs.
- Dispensing drugs.
- Storing drugs.
- Maintaining records.
- Advising patients.
- Advising other healthcare professionals.
- Responding to adverse drug reactions.
- Administering drugs/vaccines.

Who can dispense and compound prescription drugs?
Only a pharmacist or a pharmacy technician or pharmacy student working under the direct supervision of a pharmacist can perform these duties.
**Exceptions:
- RN dispensing from Health Departments and prescriber dispensing.
- There is a law in North Carolina that allows physician assistants and nurse practitioners to compound medications under direct supervision of a pharmacist.

Who may be involved in compounding and dispensing?
- Pharmacists.
- Technicians (under pharmacist supervision).
- Pharmacy Students (under pharmacist supervision).

True or False. Physician Assistants and Nurse Practitioners can legally compound medications.
True, but only under the direct supervision of a pharmacist.

How often must the pharmacist-manager be present in the pharmacy he or she manages?
Half the time the pharmacy is open or 32 hours per week, whichever is less.

If the pharmacist-manager resigns, the pharmacy will need a new permit. Can there be an interim pharmacist-manager?
Yes, another pharmacist can take on the role of the pharmacist-manager under the original permit for up to 90 days from the date the previous pharmacist-manager departed.

How many hours must the interim pharmacist-manager be present in the pharmacy he or she manages?
20 hours per week (minimum).

What must be done within 10 days of a change in the pharmacist-manager or change of owner?
An inventory of all controlled substances in the pharmacy.
Note: a record of this inventory should be kept for 3 years.

Who maintains authority and control over all keys to the pharmacy?
The pharmacist-manager.
How long can a pharmacy be open without a pharmacist being present?
90 minutes (maximum), once a pharmacist has been absent for 90 minutes or more, the pharmacy has to be closed.

Can a pharmacist serve as the pharmacist-manager for more than one pharmacy?
Most pharmacies operate under what is called a full service permit, and a pharmacist cannot be registered as the pharmacist-manager for more than one full service permit pharmacy.
Note: a pharmacist can register as the pharmacist-manager with a full service permit pharmacy and another limited service permit pharmacy (limited service permits are typically granted to locations such as nursing homes with an automated dispensing machine or volunteer pharmacies).

If a pharmacy plans to close permanently, the pharmacist-manager must notify two entities of the closing. What are these two entities?
- The Board.
- The DEA.

After the pharmacy closes, the pharmacist-manager must return the permit to the Board office within how many days?
10 days.

During what time period should a pharmacy publicly post notice of a permanent closing?
From 30 days prior to closing to 15 days after closing.

What should be done for the final 30 days of business?
Prescription files should be transferred to each customer's pharmacy of choice. Note: in the absence of specific instructions from the patient, the closing pharmacy should transfer prescription files to another pharmacy and post a notice of the transfer for 15 days after the date of closing.

Which medications should be separated from stock?
All medications that are more than 6 months out of date.

Which employee is responsible for separating these out of date medications from stock?
The pharmacist-manager.

If it is reasonably probable that a prescription contributed to the death of an individual, who must be notified?
The NCBOP.

Which employee is responsible for notifying the NCBOP of the possible event-death association and how long does this person have to make the notification?
The pharmacist-manager is responsible and should notify the NCBOP within 14 days of becoming aware of the event.

At minimum, what information must be written on a prescription order from a prescriber?
1. Date written.
2. Name and address of patient.
3. Name, address, and phone number of prescriber.
4. DEA # of prescriber (for controlled substances).
5. Name, strength, dosage form, and quantity of drug.
6. Number of refills (retail) or stop date (hospital).
7. Route of administration.
8. Directions for use.

What must be included in a pharmacy's dispensing records?
- Quantity dispensed.
- Date dispensed.
- Rx number (aka serial number).
- Identification of dispensing pharmacist.
- Refill history.
- Documentation showing that the state's requirements for drug selection were satisfied.

How long do prescriptions records have to be kept by a pharmacy?
3 years.

Does the Rx hard copy have to be held for 3 years, or is an electronic image of the prescription sufficient?
An electronically stored image of the prescription will suffice as long as a copy can be made available within 48 hours of request by the Board.
Note: when an electronic copy is stored in lieu of the hard copy, the electronic copy is considered to be the original.

Pharmacies using a computer to process prescriptions must maintain a log of signatures for pharmacists that fill/refill prescriptions each day. How long does this log have to be maintained?
3 years.

What is the signature on the log meant to indicate?
That the prescription information entered into the computer that day has been reviewed by the pharmacist and is correct.

True or false. If one uses an automated data processing system (i.e. a computer) to fill prescriptions, the computer has to be capable of printing prescription and dispensing records.
True.

Can non-controlled substance prescriptions be sent electronically or by fax from a physician office to a pharmacy?
Yes.

Can the prescriber designate someone other than himself/herself to fax or electronically send prescriptions?
Yes.

Why must all pharmacy records be stored in a readily retrievable manner?
In case the Board wishes to review, copy, or seize the records.

If the Board requests access to pharmacy records, in what time frame must the records be made available to the Board?
Within 48 hours of the request.

What is the difference between a "label" and "labeling?"
- A label functions to display the information on a drug's packaging.
- Labeling, on the other hand, includes the label, the written materials dispensed along with the prescription, and accompanying words spoken to the patient (e.g. the counseling provided by a pharmacist).

What statement must appear on the label of all prescription drugs?
"Rx only" or "Caution Federal law prohibits dispensing without a prescription."

What information must be displayed on the Rx label?
- Name of patient.
- Name and address of patient.
- Filled or dispensed by (pharmacist's name).
- Serial number (i.e. Rx number).
- Date of prescription or date of filling.
- Name of prescriber.
- Directions for use.
- Name and strength of drug.

If a brand name drug is dispensed, does the generic name also have to appear on the label?
Yes, all prescription labels must display the generic name of the drug (e.g. if brand name Lipitor® was dispensed, the generic name atorvastatin would also have to appear on the label).

Prescription labels must display the discard date of the dispensed drug. Is this the same as the expiration date?
No, the discard date is equal to one year from the dispensing date or the manufacturer's expiration date, whichever is sooner.

When labeling a stock bottle for dispensing, what must you keep in mind?
To never occlude the expiration date or storage instructions on the stock bottle, as this information must remain visible to the patient per NC pharmacy laws/rules.

Are you exposed to more liability when you dispense a pharmacist-substituted drug product?
No, there is no additional liability to pharmacists when dispensing an equivalent drug product.

What does "PRN refills" mean?
PRN refills means unlimited refills for one year from the date the Rx was written.

If the Rx was written on 10/01/12 with PRN refills and the date of first fill was 11/25/12, will the patient be able to get a refill on this Rx on 11/24/13?
No.

If the prescriber writes "PRN refills for 2 years," are the refills really valid for 2 years?
Yes, legally the prescription would be considered valid for 2 years from the date written.

What statement must be present on a veterinary prescription drug label?
"Caution: Federal law restricts this drug to use by or on the order of a licensed veterinarian."

For the products of a manufacturer to be considered eligible for use in product selection (when substitution is permitted), what does the Board require of the manufacturer?
The manufacturer must accept returns of full and partial containers of medication that are up to six (6) months beyond the labeled expiration date.

Define "equivalent drug products."
Drugs with the same generic name, active ingredient, strength, and dosage form.

What is the FDA publication that assigns a two letter code to drugs based on therapeutic equivalence evaluation findings?
The Orange Book.

What are the requirements for pharmacist-substituted generic equivalents?
The substituted generic equivalent chosen must contain the manufacturer's name on the label of the stock bottle, as well as the distributor's name, and a logo that identifies the manufacturer or distributor.

Are pharmacists required to dispense AB-rated drugs when dispensing a generic substitute?
No, not in North Carolina.

To prevent product selection, what must the prescriber do?
Sign the line that indicates the prescription should be dispensed as written.

What if the prescription blank does not have a pre-printed DAW line for the prescriber to sign on?
The prescriber can hand write "dispense as written" or "DAW" on the face of the prescription.

If a prescriber said to dispense Lipitor® in a verbal order, can you dispense atorvastatin?
Yes, for verbal orders if the prescriber does not verbalize "dispense as written," then product selection is permitted by default.

Is product selection permitted if the alternative to the written product results in a higher cost to the patient?
No, pharmacists can only dispense an equivalent drug if the **cost to the patient is lower** than the cost of the prescribed drug.

What is a narrow therapeutic index (NTI) drug?
NTI drugs are medications that walk a fine line between conferring a benefit and causing harm.

How many NTI drugs are there?
11.

What are the 11 NTI drugs?
1. Carbamazepine
2. Cyclosporine
3. Digoxin
4. Ethosuximide
5. Levothyroxine
6. Lithium
7. Phenytoin
8. Procainamide
9. Tacrolimus
10. Theophylline
11. Warfarin

Why should you know which drugs have a narrow therapeutic index?
Because it is important for the patient to consistently use the same manufacturer, as bioavailability can vary between manufacturers.

When refilling an NTI drug, can you use a manufacturer other than the one previously dispensed?
Different manufacturers can only be dispensed for refills if the prescriber and the patient give consent.
Note: document the consent.

Who is responsible for classifying drugs as NTI drugs?
The NC Secretary of Health and Human Services (HHS).

How often is the list of NTI drugs updated in North Carolina?
Every year in January, but there are rarely any changes to the list.

Can you ever dispense prescription drugs without a prescription?
No.

When you are busy, you have your technician to answer the phone and pretend to be a pharmacist. Is that legal?
No, it is illegal for someone to portray himself/herself as a pharmacist if not licensed.

Who can communicate prescription transfers?
Only pharmacists and certified technicians.

What does the transferring pharmacy have to write on the face of the prescription?
"Void"
Note: in pharmacies that process prescriptions with a computer, this step is usually taken care of by the software.

What does the transferring pharmacist or certified technician have to write on the back of the prescription?
- Name and address of pharmacy receiving the transfer.
- Name of the person giving the transfer.
- Name of the person receiving the transfer.
- Date of the transfer.

Since everything is done on a computer these days, you rarely (if ever) will have to write this information on the back of the prescription, just enter this information into the computer.

When receiving a transfer, what has to be recorded?
- Date/time of the transfer.
- Rx number assigned by the transferring pharmacy.
- Date the original Rx was written.
- Number of refills authorized on the original Rx.
- Number of refills remaining on the Rx.
- Date of last refill.
- Brand or manufacturer of the drug dispensed.
- Name and address of the transferring pharmacy.
- Name of the person giving the transfer.

For transferred prescriptions how long must the transferring & receiving pharmacy keep a copy of the Rx?
3 years from the date of last fill.

If a patient is out of refills and the pharmacist cannot obtain a refill authorization from the prescriber, what can be done?
The pharmacist can give the patient an emergency refill.

How much medication can be given in an emergency refill?
A 30-day supply (maximum).

What if the prescriber is unable to continue providing medical services to the customer?
In this case, you may give up to a 90-day supply.

Can you give multiple emergency refills?
No, they are one time only.

Can an emergency refill ever be provided for C-II drugs?
No, C-II prescriptions can never be refilled.

How much time do you have to notify the prescriber after you have dispensed an emergency refill?
72 hours.

COMPOUNDING

Are you allowed to compound something before actually getting the prescription?
Yes, as long as you are compounding based on an established pattern/prescription history.

If you compound ahead of time, but not based on an established pattern/prescription history, what is the risk?
Being classified as a manufacturer when you do not have the appropriate permit to be operating as a manufacturer.

Can you supply other pharmacies with compounded drugs for resale?
No.

If one pharmacy receives a prescription to fill, can another pharmacy fill it?
Yes, assuming they are owned by the same entity or there is a contract between the pharmacies.

Which address would have to be on the Rx label, the address of the pharmacy that received the prescription or the address of the pharmacy that filled the prescription?
The address of the pharmacy that filled the prescription.

Which pharmacy would have to keep records, the receiving pharmacy or the filling pharmacy?
Both pharmacies would have to keep records.

Do the pharmacies have to share files electronically?
Yes.

Which pharmacy would be responsible for patient consultations?
The pharmacy that received the prescription, not the pharmacy that filled the prescription.

Can a pharmacist refuse to fill a prescription?
Yes, especially if they think the Rx is fake or would cause harm.

Should a pharmacist fill a prescription if he/she knows it was written without a valid prescriber-patient relationship and a physical exam?
No, but there are exceptions.

What types of prescriptions can be written without a physical exam?
- Prescriptions for psychiatric illnesses.
- Prescriptions for the flu vaccine.
- Prescriptions for the prevention of a disease.
- Prescriptions for emergency contraceptives.
- Prescriptions for people traveling abroad.

Can a pharmacist demand photo ID before filling a prescription?
Yes.

Can a pharmacist demand photo ID before dispensing a prescription?
Yes.

What are valid forms of photo ID?
- Driver's license.
- ID card (issued by DMV).
- US passport.
- Other tamper-resistant photo ID (e.g. military ID).

Can a pharmacist refuse to fill a prescription that he/she believes is fake or illegitimate?
Yes.

Can a pharmacist refuse to fill or dispense a prescription if the customer presents an expired or fake photo ID?
Yes.

If a pharmacist refuses to fill a prescription, does this refusal get documented?
Yes, the refusal must be noted on the back of the prescription.

PHARMACY OF CHOICE

Can the prescriber choose the pharmacy?
No, the patient has the right to choose the pharmacy where their prescription(s) will be filled.

When should the offer to counsel be made?
Whenever new or transferred prescriptions are dispensed.

What type of information should a pharmacist cover during patient counseling?
- Drug name, description, and purpose.
- Dose, administration, and duration of therapy.
- Special directions for use.
- Common severe side or interactions and therapeutic contraindications that may be encountered.
  - Include how to avoid side effects and what to do if they occur.
- Techniques for self-monitoring drug therapy.
- How to properly store the medication.
- Refill information.
- What to do in the case of a missed a dose.

What vaccines/immunizations may be administered by North Carolina pharmacists?
Only vaccinations or immunizations recommended or required by the Centers for Disease Control and Prevention.

True or False. For pharmacists to give immunizations there has to be a written protocol for administration and response to adverse reactions.
True.

Pharmacists that are certified to immunize may administer vaccinations/immunizations to people of what age group?
Ages 18 and older in general, but ages 14 and older for influenza.

Which vaccines can be administered by a pharmacist in accordance with a written protocol (i.e. without consulting the individual patient's primary care provider prior to administering)?
- Influenza.
- Herpes zoster.
- Pneumococcal.
- Hepatitis B.
- Meningococcal.
- Tetanus, tetanus-diphtheria, tetanus-diphtheria-pertussis, and tetanus-diphtheria-acellular pertussis.*

*Pharmacists must not administer tetanus vaccines to patients that have an open wound, puncture, or tissue tear.

Pharmacists that administer vaccines under a written protocol with a physician must have what certification (in addition to immunization certification)?
Cardiopulmonary resuscitation (CPR) certification.

For immunizing pharmacists, how many hours of immunizing continuing education credits are required?
3 hours of CE credit every 2 years.

What information must be documented in a patient profile for pharmacist-provided immunizations?
- Name, address, and birth date of the patient.
- Date of administration.
- Administration site (e.g. right deltoid).
- Route of administration (e.g. intramuscular).
- Vaccine name, manufacturer, lot #, and expiration date.
- Dose administered.
- Name and address of patient's primary care provider.
- Name or initials of the administering pharmacist.

If the patient identifies a primary care provide (PCP), the immunizing pharmacist must notify his/her PCP within _____ after administration of any vaccination or immunization.
72 hours.

True or false. If the patient does not have a PCP, the pharmacist must direct the patient to information describing the benefits of a PCP.
True.

The information describing the benefits of a PCP must be prepared by what organization?
Any one of the following:
- North Carolina Medical Board.
- North Carolina Academy of Family Physicians.
- North Carolina Medical Society.
- Community Care of North Carolina.

When administering the influenza vaccine pursuant to a written protocol, are you required to access the North Carolina Immunization Registry prior to administration?
No, but you are required to do so for any other vaccine or immunization.

When administering any vaccine or immunization other than influenza, as described above, you must enter a record of the administration in the NC Immunization Registry within what period of time?
Within 72 hours after the administration.

Note: pharmacy records are private and there are limitations on who can gain access to the records based on the age of the patient, the problem being treated, and other legal considerations.

Who may access their pharmacy records?
- Adults (age 18 or greater) or an adult's legal guardian.
- Emancipated minors or an emancipated minor's legal guardian.
- Unemancipated minors in cases where drug therapy is for one of the following conditions:
    1. Venereal Disease.
    2. Pregnancy.
    3. Alcohol/drug abuse.
    4. Psychological diagnoses.
- The legal guardian of an unemancipated minor when the drug therapy is for a condition other than the 4 listed above.
- The issuer of the prescription.
- Another practitioner treating the patient.
- Pharmacists providing pharmacy services to the patient.
- Any person with written authorization to obtain the records signed by the patient or the patient's legal representative.
- Anyone with a subpoena, court order, or statute.
- Any business entity that provides or pays for medical care of the patient.
- An agent of the Board.
- The executor, administrator, or spouse of a deceased patient.
- Surveyors and researchers with NCBOP approval.
- The pharmacy owner or an authorized agent of the pharmacy owner.

In what circumstances should a pharmacist disclose pharmacy records?
When the pharmacist decides that such disclosure is reasonably necessary to protect the life or health of the patient/customer.

Is it a requirement for all pharmacies to have a Quality Assurance (QA) program?
Yes, QA programs are required by the Pharmacy Quality Assurance Protection Act.

Are there exceptions?
No, all pharmacies must have a QA program.

How often must the quality of a pharmacy practice be assessed?
Quality must be assessed on a continuous basis via the QA program.

What is evaluated in a pharmacy QA program?
- Quality of pharmacy services.
- Cause of errors.
    o The process of determining the cause of an error is often referred to as Root Cause Analysis (RCA).

Who responds to QA evaluations?
The pharmacy staff responds and makes recommendations for improvement.

What is the purpose of QA programs?
The purpose is to reduce medication errors.

True or False. Information from a QA program can be exploited by a manager to fire an employee.
False, no one can be punitively affected with the information provided to a QA program.

True or False. Records from a QA program are made public.
False, records from QA programs are kept confidential.

What references must be kept in the pharmacy?
- Drug equivalence references.
- Clinical drug references.
- Patient education materials.
- State and federal pharmacy statutes/rules.

Must these references be stored in paper (hard copy) form?
No, they may be stored electronically.

Are pharmacies required to have a restroom?
Yes, with hot and cold running water.

True or False. Community/Retail pharmacies are required to display the hours a pharmacist will be on duty.
True.

What are some methods a pharmacy can use to get rid of unwanted, outdated, or adulterated non-controlled substance drugs?
- Return the drugs to the manufacturer.
- Have the drugs incinerated by a permitted facility.

Note: please refer to the Federal Law Overview in the following pages for information on the disposal of unwanted controlled substances drugs.

True or False. Drugs can be donated to free clinics or pharmacies and then be dispensed to uninsured or underinsured patients.
True.

Can controlled substances be donated to a free clinic or pharmacy?
No.

Can drugs that are subject to a restricted distribution system be donated to a free clinic or pharmacy?
No.

Can compounded drugs be donated to a free clinic or pharmacy?
No.

Can biologicals be donated to a free clinic or pharmacy?
No.

Can parenteral admixtures be donated to a free clinic or pharmacy?
No.

Can drugs that require refrigeration be donated to a free clinic or pharmacy?
No.

What requirements must be met for a donated drug to be considered eligible for dispensing?
- The drug must be in the original, sealed container.
- The drug must be good for at least 6 months (i.e. at least 6 months until it expires).
- The pharmacist must conclude that the drug is not adulterated or misbranded.

Does law require donated drugs to be dispensed to eligible patients (i.e. uninsured or underinsured) at no charge?
No, a handling fee may be charged.

What packaging requirement applies to solid oral dosage forms of pseudoephedrine?
They must be packaged and sold in <u>blister packs</u>. Pseudoephedrine can never be sold as loose tablets/capsules.

What is the minimum age for purchasing pseudoephedrine?
18 years of age.

Pseudoephedrine products are required to be stored and sold from a particular location. What is this location?
Behind the pharmacy counter.

What is the maximum quantity of pseudoephedrine that can be sold to one customer in one day?
3.6 grams of pseudoephedrine total.

What is the maximum amount of pseudoephedrine that can be sold to one customer over the course of one month (30 days)?
9 grams of pseudoephedrine total.

True or False. Information about the maximum purchase quantities of pseudoephedrine must be communicated to the customer via a sign displayed in the pharmacy.
True.

True or False. The customer must provide a signature showing they agree to the limits on pseudoephedrine sales.
True.

How long does the pharmacy have to maintain records of pseudoephedrine sales?
Records must be kept for 2 years and kept in a place where they can be retrieved within 48 hours.

What are the penalties for failing to provide training for pseudoephedrine sales, failing to supervise the sale of pseudoephedrine, or failing to discipline employees for violating rules pertaining to the sale of pseudoephedrine?
- $500 fine for the first violation.
- $750 fine for the second violation.
- $1,000 fine for the third or subsequent violation.

Can you be punished for violating the reporting requirements for pseudoephedrine sales?
No.

Can you be punished for denying the sale of pseudoephedrine to customers you believe are breaking the law?
No.

Do the limits apply to pseudoephedrine products purchased pursuant to a valid prescription?
No, patients can obtain whatever amount of pseudoephedrine is indicated on the prescription, assuming the prescription is valid.

What is the definition of a drug according to the NC Controlled Substance Act (CSA)?

A drug is a substance recognized by one of the following:

- United States Pharmacopoeia (USP).
- Homeopathic Pharmacopoeia of the United States.
- National Formulary (NF).

What are the characteristics of drugs belonging to different schedules of controlled substances?

Schedule I Controlled Substance (e.g. GHB, Heroin)

- High abuse potential.
- No accepted medical use.
- Lacks safety.

Schedule II Controlled Substance (e.g. Morphine, Codeine)

- High potential for abuse.
- Accepted medical use.
- Severe potential for physical/psychological dependence.

Schedule III Controlled Substance (e.g. testosterone, dronabinol)

- Moderate abuse potential.
- Accepted medical use.
- Moderate-low potential for dependence.

Schedule IV Controlled Substance (e.g. diazepam, modafinil)

- Mild abuse potential.
- Accepted medical use.
- Mild potential for physical/psychological dependence.

Schedule V Controlled Substance

- Low abuse potential.
- Accepted medical use.
- Low potential for physical/psychological dependence.
- May be sold in NC without a prescription.
    - Must be sold by licensed pharmacist.
    - Customer must furnish suitable identification.
    - The customer's name and address as well as the name and quantity of product sold should be recorded.
    - Customer must be 18 years of age or older.
    - Pharmacist must be satisfied that the customer is buying the drug for a medical purpose; otherwise, the pharmacist may refuse the sale of the drug.

<u>Schedule VI (e.g. Marijuana)</u>
- Relatively low abuse potential.
- No accepted medical use or need for further study.
- Relatively low potential for dependence.

Who is responsible for maintaining inventory records for controlled substances?
Manufacturers → Distributers → Dispensers (Pharmacies).

Note: essentially, everyone that is involved with controlled substances must maintain inventory records.

When a new pharmacist-manager is appointed, what has to be done with the controlled substances in the pharmacy?
An inventory of all controlled substances has to be taken within 10 days.

What form is required for ordering C-II drugs?
DEA Form 222 is required for distribution of C-II drugs.
Note: the same form is also used for ordering C-I drugs.

Can a C-II prescription ever be given to the pharmacy verbally (i.e. over the telephone) by a physician's secretary?
No, a written prescription is required for C-II medications and prescriptions for C-II medications must be hand signed (electronic and stamped signatures are not valid).
**Exception: in "emergency situations" a prescriber (the actual prescriber, not a nurse or secretary representing the prescriber) may verbally order a C-II prescription.
- The pharmacist must reduce the verbal prescription to writing immediately.
- The emergency prescription must be only in a quantity necessary to treat the patient for the emergency period, not to exceed a 72 hour supply.

Are faxed C-II prescriptions ever considered valid?
Only if written for the following patient populations:
- Hospice.
- Long term care.
- Home infusion.

Can a prescription for a C-II medication ever be refilled?
No, refills are not allowed on C-II medications.

Use of preprinted prescription blanks is _____ for schedule II through V controlled substances.
Prohibited.

In NC, Schedule II and III Synthetic Cannabinoids (dronabinol and nabilone) can only be used legally as what?
Antiemetics for cancer patients undergoing chemotherapy.
**Point of confusion: 10A NCAC 26E .0305 still says that both nabilone and dronabinol are Schedule II controlled substances; however, the DEA reclassified dronabinol as a Schedule III controlled substance in 1999.
Note: dronabinol is in fact a Schedule III controlled substance.

In what ways can a pharmacy receive prescriptions for C-III and C-IV prescriptions?
- Written.
- Verbal.
- Faxed.

At most, how many refills can a prescriber authorize (at one time) for C-III and C-IV prescriptions?
5 refills.

How long are C-III and C-IV prescriptions valid?
6 months from the date written.

When prescriptions are given to a pharmacy verbally, what must the person receiving the prescription do?
Reduce the verbal prescription to writing immediately.

Do C-V prescriptions have any of the limitations we see with C-II, C-III or C-IV prescriptions?
No, C-V prescriptions do not expire after six months and they can be refilled under the same rules as non-controlled substances.

A patient requests a copy of their controlled substance prescription. Should you give the patient a copy?
Legally, you may give the patient a copy of the prescription, but if you do you must write on the face of the copy "COPY - FOR INFORMATION ONLY."
Note: you can also choose to deny their request, use your professional judgment.

What special requirement is there for free samples of medications?
Free samples of controlled substances can only be given upon written request.
Note: a record of written requests must be maintained by the manufacturer for 2 years.

True or False. It is fine to fill a prescription that you know has been obtained through misrepresentation (e.g. you know that the patient faked an illness to obtain a medication).
False.

A patient insists that you dispense 60 tablets of his controlled substance medication, but the doctor wrote for 30 tablets with 2 refills. Is there any way you can dispense 60 tablets?

Only if you receive authorization from the doctor to dispense more than the written quantity, the same would be true for psychiatric medications.
Note: document the conversation on the prescription hard copy (i.e. Okay to dispense #60 per Dr. Jones on 5/31/13 and your signature or initials).

Bob has the following prescription: Xanax 1 mg, 1 PO QD, # 30 with 5 Refills written 5/30/13. Bob purchased 15 tablets 6 times (the initial fill plus 5 refills). Bob is due for another refill on 9/18/13, is he able to get this refill (refill #6)?
Note: C-IV drugs can only have 5 refills in 6 months

Yes, the important point is that you do not dispense more than the total amount authorized in the prescription (in this case 180 tablets), not how many fills the prescription has been divided into.

Is there a days supply limit on Schedule II controlled substances?

No, please see the January 2008 NCBOP Newsletter (first page, top right column) for further explanation.
Note:
- Physician Assistants and Nurse Practitioners are limited to a 30-day supply per fill for C-II and C-III prescriptions.
- There is a helpful summary of prescribing limitations for midlevel practitioners (a one-page PDF) on ncbop.org under "Physician Assistants/Nurse Practitioners" in the "Pharmacist FAQs."

Which medications require a photo ID for pickup?
- Schedule II medications.
- Combination Schedule III medications (e.g. Norco).

What are acceptable forms of photo ID?
- Driver's license.
- Identification card issued by the NC DMV.
- Military identification.
- Passport.

What must be recorded during the transaction when selling C-II or combination C-III prescriptions?
- Date of sale.
- Rx number.
- Customer's name.
- Type of photo ID presented (e.g. passport).
- Photo ID number (e.g. driver's license number).

How long must you keep records from C-II and combination C-III prescription sales?
3 years.

Is it okay if the customer uses an expired photo ID?
No, the photo ID is not considered valid if it is expired.

Someone wants to pick-up a prescription for fentanyl patches. The person hands you a Mexico driver's license. Can you accept this photo ID?
Yes, valid/unexpired driver's licenses, passports, and military IDs from any state or country are acceptable as long as there is a photo, an expiration date, and an ID number.

A patient wants to pick-up a prescription for generic Lortab. When you ask the patient for a photo ID, they state that they do not have one. What option can you give the individual?
If the patient does not have an acceptable photo ID, they can get someone else with a valid ID to pickup the prescription for them.

Can medical devices and/or drugs be sold without a permit?
No.

Why was the North Carolina Controlled Substance Reporting System (NCCSRS) established?
Because of prescription drug overdose deaths in North Carolina.

What is the most common cause of overdose death in NC?
Unintentional opioid overdose.

What medication is associated with a high rate of overdose death?
Methadone used in the treatment of severe pain.

What is the NCCSRS meant to accomplish?
- Identify patients abusing controlled substances.
- Prevent diversion of controlled substances.
- Prevent unintentional drug overdoses.
- Reduce investigation costs in cases involving Rx drugs.

When must pharmacies submit controlled substance dispensing information to the NCCSRS?
Information from controlled substance dispensing must be reported to the NCCSRS within 3 business days after delivering (i.e. dispensing) a controlled substance prescription; however, dispensers are encouraged to report the information within 24 hours of delivery.
Note: for controlled substance prescriptions that do not exceed a 48-hour supply, NCCSRS reporting is not required.

Is information from NCCSRS made available to the public?
No, this information is confidential.

How long is information stored in the NCCSRS?
Information is kept in the NCCSRS for 6 years then purged.

True or False. Health facilities (e.g. hospitals, nursing homes) that practice pharmacy must obtain a permit from the NCBOP.
True.

In what circumstances does a decentralized pharmacy (e.g. a hospital satellite pharmacy) require a separate permit to practice pharmacy?
1. Dispensing is primarily to outpatients.
2. Inventory is obtained from a source outside of the health facility.
3. Pharmacy management is not supervised by the central pharmacy.

What type of professional must hold the position of director of a health care facility pharmacy?
A licensed pharmacist.
Note: in the North Carolina laws and rules, the director of a health care facility pharmacy is referred to as the "pharmacist-manager."

What are the pharmacist-manager's responsibilities in a hospital or health care facility setting?
1. Provide policies and procedures.
   a. For safe/effective drug distribution.
   b. For compounding.
   c. For labeling.
   d. For educating/training pharmacy and nursing employees that prepare IV admixtures.
   e. For acquiring and disposing of drugs that are expired, recalled, misbranded or unusable.
   f. For handling and storing drugs and devices.
   g. Monthly inspections of areas where drugs are stored/dispensed/administered (quarterly inspections for LTC facilities).
   h. For drug samples.
   i. For patient's home medications.
2. Specify how drug products will be acquired.
3. Help create a drug formulary.
4. Ensure all drugs are prepared, packed and labeled appropriately.
5. Certify that dispensing is done only by those deemed legal to dispense (i.e. pharmacists).
6. Supervise pharmacy department employees.
7. Keep records necessary to make sure patient health is not endangered.
8. Review discrepancies with controlled substance counts within 24 hours of discovery.
9. Report significant losses of controlled substance to the NCBOP and DEA.

Are there specific physical requirements for a health care facility pharmacy (e.g. pharmacy must be at least 200 sq ft)?
No, the space allocated for the pharmacy just has to be sufficient, sanitary, well-lit and enclosed.

Are there specific equipment requirements (e.g. the pharmacy must have graduated cylinders)?
No, the pharmacy just has to be equipped with sufficient equipment for drug compounding, dispensing and storage.

Administration of drugs/immunizations falls under the scope of pharmacy practice. Do health facilities that only participate in the practice of pharmacy to the extent that they administer drugs and immunizations need to obtain a permit from the NCBOP?
No (this is the only exception).

In hospitals with 24-hour outpatient pharmacies, is it required for all outpatient controlled substance dispensing (including emergency room) be done by the pharmacy?
Yes, if the hospital does not have a 24-hour outpatient pharmacy and the pharmacy is closed, dispensing can take place from the ER in accordance with a pharmacist-designed system for dispensing.
Note:
- Formulary of controlled substances is developed by the ER committee and the hospital pharmacy.
- Dispensing is limited to a 24-hour supply.
- Dispensing records must be checked by a pharmacist for correctness on a weekly basis (at minimum).

In a hospital without a 24-hour pharmacy, how do patients get drugs and pharmaceutical care?
Patients get pharmacy services from and on-call pharmacist, and drugs can be obtained from an ancillary drug cabinet.

Do ancillary drug cabinets have to be locked?
Yes.

How many doses of a drug can be kept in these cabinets?
Up to 5 doses of any drug approved for storage in an ancillary drug cabinet.

How is removal of inventory from these cabinets tracked?
Movement of inventory through the ancillary drug cabinet is tracked using the "record of withdrawal."

How long is the pharmacy required to keep the record of withdrawal used for ancillary drug cabinets?
3 years.

Can a nurse dispense drugs instead of an on-call pharmacist when the pharmacy is closed?
Only if the nurse has been trained by the pharmacist-manager to dispense; however, the nurse still cannot dispense certain restricted medications without a pharmacist.

In a health care facility <u>with</u> a 24-hour pharmacy, can nurses dispense?
No, in this case all dispensing must be done by a pharmacist.

Can non-pharmacists dispense from an ER?
Only if the facility's pharmacy is closed.
Note: in facilities with a 24-hour pharmacy, all dispensing must be done by a pharmacist.

Which drugs may be dispensed by the ER?
Drugs on the ER formulary.

Who decides which drugs are on the ER formulary?
The pharmacist-manager in conjunction with a committee from the ER.

Who packages and labels drugs for ER dispensing?
Drugs are pre-packaged and pre-labeled by a pharmacist.

ER dispensing records must be kept for how long?
3 years.

In a health care facility, what department is responsible for maintaining dispensing records?
Pharmacy.

If a patient is given drug samples, is this activity recorded in the dispensing records?
Yes.

True or False. Repackaging drugs in a health care facility is against the law.
False, many hospitals purchase drugs in bulk bottles, and then repackage the drugs into unit doses.
Note: The benefit to unit dose packaging is that each dose (e.g. each tablet) can have its own sealed package and label with information (e.g. drug name, strength, NDC, expiration, lot number).

Is dispensing of starter packs included in dispensing records?
Yes, at this point you should be able to see that basically any medication given to a patient should be recorded in the dispensing records.

Can medication orders in a hospital be signed electronically by the prescriber?
Yes, the orders can be signed or verified electronically by the prescriber.

If patient health depends on how quickly a particular drug is given, can that drug be stored on the patient care unit?
Yes, but no more than 5 doses of any one drug can be kept on the patient care unit.

Morphine was prepared for a patient, but the patient refused the dose. Can the nurse destroy the drug immediately?
Yes, but only if witnessed by another health care provider.
Note: the destruction would have to be documented and the witness would have to sign off on the documentation.

In a health care facility, can automated dispensing devices (e.g. Pyxis® machines) be utilized?
Yes.

Who determines the specific contents of an emergency kit?
The pharmacist-manager in conjunction with medical staff.
Note: pharmacist-managers can delegate this responsibility.

What types of drugs can be included in an emergency kit?
Drugs that need to be administered quickly in order to have an optimal effect on the patient (e.g. epinephrine).

When can emergency kits be used?
In emergencies only.

How often does an emergency kit have to be inspected for expired medications?
Every 30 days (every 90 days in the case of LTC facilities).

Who is responsible for checking stock for expired drugs?
A pharmacist or someone appointed by a pharmacist.
Note: a pharmacist usually appoints a technician to do this.

When checking for expired medications in an emergency kit, one should also verify that the _____ on the kit is in-tact.
Seal.

Does there need to be a physician's order to use drugs from an emergency kit?
Yes.

If an emergency kit is used, what department has to be informed and why?
Pharmacy, so they can restock the emergency kit.

Does a pharmacy have to maintain records of all transactions involving controlled substances?
Yes, for 3 years.

How are technicians and pharmacists held responsible for what they compound and dispense in a health care facility?
Through compounding and dispensing records which identify those involved in the compounding and dispensing process.

How long do these records have to be maintained?
30 days.

Who is responsible for documenting medication errors?
The pharmacist-manager.

How long do you maintain medication error records?
3 years.

Upon request from the NCBOP, how quickly must a pharmacy make the requested records available?
Within 48 hours.

What are some examples of an automated medication system?
Pyxis®, AccuDose®, Omnicell®, & ROBOT-Rx®.

In each facility that utilizes them, who is responsible for oversight of automated medication systems?
The Multidisciplinary Committee for Decentralized Automated Medication Systems.

Who creates the Multidisciplinary Committee for Decentralized Automated Medication Systems?
The pharmacist-manager.

Is anyone in particular required to be on the multidisciplinary committee?
Yes, the pharmacist-manager, or his/her designee, is required to be on the committee.

Who can stock or restock an automated medication system?
- Pharmacists.
- Pharmacy technicians supervised by a pharmacist.

Note: registered nurses may stock and restock systems equipped with bar code verification, electronic verification, or a similar verification process is utilized.

How do pharmacists ensure that the right drug is being placed in the automated medication system?
By adhering to one of the following procedures:
- Conduct and document daily audits (i.e. inspect random samplings) of drugs that have been, or will be, placed into the system by pharmacy technicians.
- For systems that utilize bar code verification (or similar technology), conduct quarterly quality assurance reviews.

In settings where an automated dispensing system is utilized to dispense patient-specific unit doses, do pharmacists have to review each medication selected and labeled by the system?
Pharmacists only have to review/approve the initial fill, subsequent fills do not require a pharmacist's review/approval.

What records specific to automated medication systems need to be maintained?
- Daily (or quarterly) audits of stocking or restocking.
- Daily audits of centralized automated medication system output.
- Transaction records for all non-controlled medications.
- Transaction records for all controlled substances.
- Reports related to the quality assurance program.
- Reports regarding who has access to the system.

Drugs stored in an automated dispensing device must be reviewed ____.
Monthly.

Before drugs from an automated dispensing device are made available to a nurse, what must be done with the drug order?
A *prospective* drug utilization review by a pharmacist (e.g. check the dose, screen for allergies and drug interactions).
Note: drugs classified as "override medications" by the Multidisciplinary Committee for Decentralized Automated Medication Systems are subject to a *retrospective* drug utilization review by a pharmacist.

For filling floor stock and unit dose dispensing systems, can a technician check another technician's work?
Yes, as long as they are a Validating Technician.

What qualifications are required of Validating Technicians?
- Certified technician registered with the NCBOP.
- Associate's degree in pharmacy technology.
- Completed training as determined by the pharmacist-manager.

REMOTE ORDER ENTRY

May a pharmacy outsource its order entry work?
Yes, remote order entry is legal, as long as the pharmacy doing the order entry is under same ownership or there is a contract between the pharmacies.

Do remote order entry pharmacists require special training?
Yes, they must be trained on the relevant policies/procedures of the pharmacy outsourcing the work.

Who has to store information from remotely entered orders?
The entity that is actually dispensing the medications.

If pharmacists are entering orders for North Carolina remotely from out-of-state, do they have to hold an active North Carolina license?
Yes.

What are some of the key points from the rules pertaining to clinical pharmacist practitioners (CPP)?

- Application fee is $100.
    - Application and fee are submitted to the NCBOP and then forwarded to the Medical Board.
- Renewal few is $50.
    - Renewal is annually on the birthday of the CPP.
    - Grace period for renewal is 30 days.
- Must earn 35 hours of CE credit annually.
    - This is 20 additional hours of CE in addition to the standard 15 hours required for all pharmacists.
    - Maintain documentation of CE at practice site.
- Can modify drug doses, dosing schedules, dosage forms, and order labs.
- Can implement drug therapy according to a signed, written protocol with a physician.
- Need a DEA number to prescribe controlled substances.
- Are comparable to a physician assistant or a nurse practitioner.

What combinations of education, certification, and experience qualify one to register with the Board as a CPP?

Combination #1:
- Unrestricted NC pharmacist license.
- Board of Pharmaceutical Specialties (BPS) certification, Certified Geriatric Pharmacist, or completion of an ASHP-accredited residency including 2 years of clinical experience.

Combination #2:
- Unrestricted NC pharmacist license.
- Doctor of Pharmacy degree.
- 3 years of clinical experience.
- NCCPC or ACPE certification in 1 area of practice which is covered by the CPP agreement.

Combination #3:
- Unrestricted NC pharmacist license.
- Bachelor of Science in Pharmacy.
- 5 years of clinical experience.
- NCCPC or ACPE certification in 2 areas of practice, at least one of which is an area of practice covered by the CPP agreement.

How many clinical pharmacist practitioners can be supervised by one physician?
3 (maximum).

Clinical pharmacist practitioners can be reprimanded by what professional boards?
- The Board of Pharmacy.
- The Medical Board.

Are ID badges optional for healthcare professionals?
No, healthcare professionals must wear an ID badge when providing patient care, which has to display the professional's name and the credential they hold (e.g. John Smith, PharmD).

Are there exceptions to wearing an ID badge?
Yes, a badge is not required if the practitioner's name is prominently displayed in the office.

In what setting may a registered nurse (RN) dispense medications?
Health department clinics.

How do these nurses know how to dispense?
They complete training in labeling and packaging.

Are RNs limited to dispensing only certain drugs?
Yes, they can only dispense drugs listed on a formulary from the Department of Health and Human Services.

What types of drugs are typically on the health department formulary for RN dispensing?
- Anti-tuberculosis drugs.
- Antibiotics for treating STDs.
- Contraceptives for pregnancy prevention.
- Vitamin and mineral supplements.
- Topical drugs for certain conditions.
  - Lice.
  - Scabies.
  - Impetigo.
  - Diaper rash.
  - Vaginitis.

Can a health department formulary for RN dispensing include controlled substances?
No.

True or False. Health departments with dispensing RNs must hold a pharmacy permit.
True.

Are there special policy/procedure requirements for RN dispensing?
Yes, there has to be written, Board-approved procedures for storage, packaging, labeling, and delivery of prescriptions.

Is pharmacist involvement required at all?
Yes, dispensing records have to be reviewed at least weekly by a pharmacist, and a pharmacist must be available at least once weekly to provide consultations.

What about a pharmacist in charge (PIC)?
There must be a pharmacist responsible for all dispensing activities at the health department where RNs are dispensing.

Can nurse practitioners (NP) and physician's assistants (PA) dispense drugs they prescribe?
Yes.

If NP or PA dispensing takes place, does the facility need a pharmacy permit?
Yes.

Can this process take place without pharmacist involvement?
No, a pharmacist must:
- Be available for consultations (may be done via telephone).
- Pre-package/pre-label all drugs.
- Perform a weekly retrospective review of all dispensing.

How does one obtain a nuclear pharmacy permit?
Submit an application to the Board certifying that he/she is a currently licensed pharmacist with nuclear pharmacist qualifications.

What are the qualifications for becoming a nuclear pharmacist?
Has obtained Board of Pharmaceutical Specialties (BPS) certification as a nuclear pharmacist, or meets minimum standards for "authorized user status."

What are the minimum standards for obtaining "authorized user status?"
- Obtain 200 contact hours of instruction in nuclear pharmacy and radioactive material safety and use from an approved college of pharmacy.
- Obtain 500 hours of clinical nuclear pharmacy training under a certified nuclear pharmacist.

Are there any special physical requirements for a nuclear pharmacy?
Yes, there needs to be a storage and product decay area that provides radioactivity protection to all areas around the pharmacy. In fact, before the Board will grant a permit to a nuclear pharmacy, floor plans must be submitted to the Board.

True or False. Use of a tamper-evident seal prior to dispensing radiopharmaceuticals is recommended but not required.
False, tamper-evident seals are required on radiopharmaceutical prescriptions.

If a radiopharmaceutical product is returned to the pharmacy with a broken seal, can it be re-used?
No, if the tamper-evident seal is broken, then the container and the contents of the container must be considered contaminated.

What cautionary statement must be displayed on the label of all radiopharmaceutical materials?
"Caution: Radioactive Materials"

Are there any special symbols that must be displayed on the label of all radiopharmaceutical materials?
Yes, the standard radiation symbol.

What other information must appear on the label of a radiopharmaceutical prescription?

- Name of the pharmaceutical and radionuclide dispensed.
- Chemical form of the radiopharmaceutical dispensed.
- Amount of radioactivity of the radiopharmaceutical and the exact time the radioactivity was measured.
- Exact time of expiration of the dispensed product.
- For liquid products, the volume dispensed.
- For solid products, the number of capsules or weight of the dispensed product.
- For products in the gaseous phase, the number of ampules, vials, or syringes in the dispensed product.
- Pharmacy name, address and telephone number.
- Prescription number or lot number.

What are the special equipment requirements for pharmacies dispensing compounded sterile products?

- Devices that create Class 100 conditions in the work area where critical sites are exposed and critical activities are performed.
- A sink with hot and cold running water near the compounding area for hand scrubbing.
- Disposal containers (e.g. sharps containers, cytotoxic waste containers).
- Biohazard cabinets for cytotoxic drugs.
- Refrigerators and freezers equipped with thermometers.
- Temperature-controlled delivery containers.
- Infusion devices (if needed).

What supplies must be maintained in the inventory of pharmacies that dispense compounded sterile products?

- Needles.
- Syringes.
- Disinfectant solution.
- Bactericidal soap.
- Lint-free disposable towels/wipes.
- Filters.
- Cytotoxic drug spill kit.
- Disposable masks, caps, gowns, and gloves.

What reference materials must be available in pharmacies that dispense compounded sterile products?

- ASHP Handbook of Injectable Drugs.
- King's Guide to Parenteral Admixtures.
- American Hospital Formulary Service.
- ASHP Procedures for Handling Cytotoxic Drugs.

What special knowledge must a pharmacist-manager have for a pharmacy that dispenses compounded sterile products?

- Compounding and dispensing sterile products.
- Principles of aseptic technique.
- Principles of quality assurance.

What are the pharmacist-manager responsibilities in a setting where compounded sterile products are dispensed?

- Develop and review policies and procedures.
- Develop and review training manuals.
- Develop and review quality assurance programs.
- Assure there is a system for disposing of infectious waste that does not endanger public health.
- Maintain reports that insure patient health, safety, and welfare for 3 years.

What must appear on the label of compounded sterile products?
- Instructions for storage to maintain sterility.
- Warning labels for oncology drugs.

What are the additional requirements for pharmacies that prepare anti-neoplastic drugs?
- Class II vertical airflow biological safety cabinet (or something similar) with strict cleaning procedures.
- Disposable gloves and gowns with tight cuffs.
- Safety and containment techniques for compounding.
- Disposal procedures in compliance with all laws.
- Spills clean-up procedures.
- Shipping procedures that minimize the risk of rupturing the container.

In terms of compounded sterile products, what is meant by "quality assurance?"
Assuring that the pharmacy is capable of consistently meeting sterility specifications with the products they compound.

What must be included in the quality assurance procedures for pharmacies that compound sterile products?
- Recall procedures.
- Storage and dating of products.
- Maintenance of refrigerator/freezer temperature logs.
- Maintenance and report of laminar air flow hood certification.
- Regular replacement of pre-filters for clean air sources with documentation of dates pre-filters are replaced.
- End-product testing for microbial contamination with documentation of the testing.
- Justification/references validating the choice of expiration dates given to compounded products.
- Regular quality assurance audits that include infection control and aseptic technique audits.

Is there a rule in NC that says pharmacists cannot dispense at such a high rate that it poses a threat to public health?
Yes.

If a pharmacist asks a prescriber to switch drug therapy, are there any disclosures that the pharmacist must make?
Yes, the pharmacist must disclose any relationships with the drug manufacturer of the drug they are requesting.

What is the maximum consecutive number of hours that a pharmacy permit holder can require a pharmacist to work?
12 hours per day.

Are pharmacists entitled to a lunch break?
Yes, if a pharmacist works more than six (6) consecutive hours in a day, they are entitled to a 30 minute lunch break and another 15 minutes break.

What special requirement applies to written prescriptions that are being billed to NC Medicaid?
All written prescriptions billed to NC Medicaid must be on tamper-resistant prescription pads.
Note: this does not apply to e-prescriptions, faxed prescriptions, or verbal prescriptions.

A prescription is written for 30 tablets with 5 refills. Can the pharmacist dispense more than 30 tablets to the patient?
Yes, unless the prescription is for a controlled substance or a psychiatric medication, in which case authorization would need to be obtained from the prescriber.
Note: physician assistants and nurse practitioners can only write for 30 days per fill on C-II and C-III controlled substances.

During a state of emergency or disaster, does insurance have to pay for early refills or to replace prescriptions filled?
Yes, insurance plans must allow for one refill that would otherwise be considered too soon to refill.
Note: if no refills remain, then the insurance must pay for one replacement fill.

What conditions must be met for a patient to qualify for the early refill or replacement prescription?
- A state of emergency or disaster has been declared.
- The patient resides in the area involved.
- The Rx is requested by the patient within 29 days of the start of the emergency/disaster.

True or False. A prescription insurance plan must give all pharmacies (within an area) the chance to participate in their plan before providing coverage to patients.
True.

Your cousin wants to change the name of her candy store to "The Candy Apothecary." Can she do that?
No, certain terms (listed below) cannot be displayed in advertisements/signage without first registering with the NCBOP as a pharmacy.
- Drug.
- Pharmacy.
- Prescription.
- Prescription drugs.
- Rx.
- Apothecary.

Why does the NCBOP prohibit non-registered entities from using those terms?
Because those terms imply that the advertising entity is legally registered to practice pharmacy.

FEDERAL PHARMACY LAW
OVERVIEW

What is a "misbranded" drug?
Many things can be construed as misbranding. Below is a list of some examples of misbranding:
- False or misleading labeling.
- Noncompliant packaging/labeling.
- Unclear wording on the label.
- Inadequate directions for use.
- Drug poses a danger if used as prescribed.
- Generic name is not displayed in font at least half as large as the brand name font.

What is an "adulterated" drug?
A drug that has a quality, strength, or purity that is different from what is stated on the label.

Federal law states that a prescriber submitting an oral emergency order for a C-II prescription must furnish the dispensing pharmacy with a written and signed prescription hard copy within 7 days. North Carolina law does not specify the timeframe in which the prescriber must furnish a hard copy. So, is the prescriber required to furnish the hard copy within 7 days or not?
In cases where federal law and state law do not match, you are expected to follow the law that is stricter (in this case, federal law). So, when a prescriber submits an oral emergency order for a C-II, he/she must furnish the dispensing pharmacy with a written and signed hard copy within 7 days.

What were the shortcomings of the Pure Food and Drug Act of 1906?
- Only purity was addressed.
  - Safety was not addressed.
  - Therapeutic false claims were not prohibited.

What historical event led to the Food, Drug, and Cosmetic Act of 1938 (FDCA)?
The sulfanilamide disaster, in which over 100 people died from using an elixir of sulfanilamide dissolved in diethylene glycol (i.e. antifreeze).

What impact did the Food, Drug, and Cosmetic Act of 1938 have on pharmacy?
This legislation required drug manufacturers to prove the safety of a drug via a New Drug Application (NDA) before being allowed to sell it.

What did the Durham-Humphrey Amendment (1951) accomplish?
Led to the creation of 2 drug categories:
- Over-the-counter (OTC).
- Prescription/Legend (Rx).

Note: this amendment also required Rx drugs to have the words, "Caution Federal law prohibits dispensing without a prescription" on the label.

What was a major effect of the Kefauver-Harris Amendment (1962)?
Evidence of effectiveness must be provided by drug manufacturers before a drug can be sold.

What rules come from the Controlled Substance Act of 1970?
- Records for controlled substances must be kept separate from other prescription records.
- You can only do a partial fill for Schedule II drugs if the remainder can be filled within 72 hours.
  - If partial fill was given, but remainder cannot be filled within 72 hours, prescriber must be notified.
- Schedule III, IV, and V drugs can be transferred to another pharmacy only one time.
  Note: transfers are unlimited for pharmacies that share a real-time, online database.

How did the Poison Prevention Packaging Act of 1970 change the way we dispense drugs?
This act requires drugs to be dispensed in child-resistant packaging (one exception is nitroglycerin sublingual tablets).

What does the Prescription Drug Marketing Act of 1987 say?
You cannot sell, buy, or trade drug samples.
Note: violation can result in a $250,000 fine and a 10-year prison sentence.

How did the Omnibus Reconciliation Act of 1990 (OBRA '90) change pharmacy practice?

By requiring drug utilization reviews (DUR) and pharmaceutical care (i.e. pharmacist counseling) for Medicaid patients.

What is the purpose of the Health Insurance Portability and Accountability Act of 1996 (HIPAA)?

To keep protected health information (PHI) confidential and secure.

How did the Food and Drug Administration Modernization Act of 1997 change prescription labeling?

This act allowed the statement "Caution Federal law prohibits dispensing without a prescription" to be reduced to "Rx only."

State Board of Pharmacy
Each state has its own board of pharmacy which is responsible for protecting the health, safety, and welfare of its citizens in matters related to pharmacy. This is accomplished through the enforcement of state & federal pharmacy laws, rules, and regulations.

Food and Drug Administration (FDA)
The FDA enforces drug manufacturing laws and regulates prescription drug advertising, which is known as "direct to consumer" (DTC) advertising.

Drug Enforcement Agency (DEA)
The DEA enforces of the Federal Controlled Substance Act, and determines which drugs are placed on the federal controlled substance schedule.

Occupational Safety and Health Administration (OSHA)
OSHA enforces health and safety laws. The most important topic OSHA deals with in pharmacy is minimizing the risk of employee exposure to bloodborne pathogens. This is particularly relevant to pharmacies that compound infusions and/or administer vaccinations.

Federal Trade Commission (FTC)
The FTC is in charge of regulating advertisement of OTC drugs, medical devices, cosmetics, and foods.
Note: Vitamins and herbal supplements are considered to be "food" in the eyes of the law.

Class I Recalls
A recall is categorized as class I if there is a reasonable probability that use of (or exposure to) the recalled product will cause serious adverse health consequences up to and including death.

Class II Recalls
A recall is categorized as class II if there is a possibility that use of (or exposure to) the recalled product could cause temporary or medically reversible adverse health consequences.

Class III Recalls
A recall is categorized as class III if use of the recalled product is unlikely to cause adverse health consequences.

Review Question:
What is the most serious class of FDA recall?
Class I recall.

True or false. Schedule I controlled substances can be dispensed pursuant to a valid, hand-signed prescription.
False, Schedule I controlled substances have no accepted medical use and cannot be prescribed.

In what setting might you find Schedule I controlled substances?
The only place Schedule I controlled substances can be legally utilized is in a legitimate research laboratory registered with the DEA to use Schedule I controlled substances.

True or false. Schedule II controlled substance prescription records can be stored in the same file as other prescription medications.
False, Schedule II prescription records must be stored separately from all other prescription records.

After an initial inventory of controlled substances has been taken (e.g. when the pharmacy first opens for business), how frequently must an inventory of controlled substances be taken?
At least every two years.

When taking an inventory of controlled substances, does the law require you to account for drug samples?
Yes, drug samples that contain controlled substances must be accounted for in the inventory record.

When Schedule II controlled substances are sent to a reverse distributor because they are expired, damaged, or otherwise unusable, what form should be used?
DEA Form 222.

Who would be responsible for filling out the Form 222?
The reverse distributor – the entity receiving the substance is always the one that fills out the form.

When Schedule III – V controlled substances are returned, is a DEA Form 222 necessary?
No, Schedule III – V controlled substances may be transferred using only an invoice (a DEA Form 222 is only used for Schedule I and II controlled substances).

According to <u>federal</u> law, how long are pharmacies required to keep controlled substance return records, prescription records, and inventory records?
2 years.

True or false. Federal law prohibits e-prescribing of C-II drugs.
False, federal law permits e-prescribing of C-II through C-V controlled substance & non-controlled substance prescriptions.

According to federal law, C-II prescriptions must be filled within how many days after being signed by the prescriber?
Federal law places no time limit within which a C-II prescription must be filled (i.e. the prescription is considered valid for an unlimited period of time after it is issued). Note, however, that North Carolina law now imposes 6-month expiration on all C-II prescriptions. This new law became effective October 1, 2013. All C-II prescriptions written on or after October 1, 2013 are subject to 6-month expiration.

True or false. For controlled substance prescriptions, the maximum quantity that can be dispensed according to *federal law* is a 30-days' supply.
False, although some states and some insurance carriers limit controlled substance quantities to a 30-day supply, there are no specific federal limits.

Are verbal/oral orders for C-II controlled substances permitted?
Only in emergency situations.
Note: quantity prescribed must be <u>limited</u> to the amount adequate to treat the patient for the duration of the emergency period, up to a 72-hour supply.

After calling in an emergency C-II prescription, what must the prescriber do next?
Provide the pharmacy with a written and signed hard copy, which the pharmacy attaches to and files with the verbal order.

When emergency C-II prescriptions are called in, a prescriber has how many days to furnish the pharmacy with a written/signed prescription?
7 days according to federal law.

True or false. Refills for C-II prescriptions are permitted by federal law (up to 5 refills in 6 months).
False, refills for <u>C-II</u> prescriptions are prohibited by federal law.

There are three exceptions which allow for C-II facsimile prescriptions to serve as the original prescription, what are they?
1. The prescription is being compounded for <u>home infusion</u>.
2. The prescription is for a patient in a <u>long-term care facility</u>.
3. The prescription is for a patient enrolled in a <u>hospice care program</u>.

Can a prescriber post-date a prescription for a controlled substance (e.g. record the date of issuance as 8/14 when he/she actually wrote the prescription in 8/12)?
No, the prescription must be dated for the day it is signed.

Can a controlled substance be delivered or shipped to an individual in another country if it is dispensed pursuant to a valid prescription?
No, exportation of a controlled substance in this manner is prohibited by the federal controlled substances act.

Prescribers that want to prescribe Schedule III – V controlled substances for treatment of narcotic addiction (i.e. buprenorphine) must display what piece of additional information on the face of the prescription?
Their unique DEA registration identification number that begins with an "X" which is granted to prescribers that have obtained the necessary waiver* from the DEA (in addition to their standard DEA registration number).

> *Typically, controlled substances used to treat narcotic addiction can only be prescribed, administered, and/or dispensed from within a Narcotic Treatment Facility (NTF), but the DEA can grant a waiver to prescribers allowing them to prescribe, administer, and/or dispense C-III through C-V drugs for treatment of narcotic addiction outside of a NTF.

What should be done in the event that theft or loss of a controlled substance is discovered?
The DEA should be notified upon discovery of the theft/loss and a DEA Form 106 should be completed to document the theft/loss.

Summary of Federal Controlled Substance Act Requirements

	Schedule II	Schedule III & IV	Schedule V
DEA Registration	Required	Required	Required
Receiving Records	DEA Form-222	Invoices	Invoices
Prescriptions	Written/Electronic*	Written/ Electronic, Oral, or Faxed	Written/ Electronic, Oral, Faxed, or Over The Counter**
Refills	No	No more than 5 within 6 months	As authorized when prescription is issued
Distribution Between Registrants	DEA Form-222	Invoices	Invoices
Theft or Significant Loss	Report and complete DEA Form 106	Report and complete DEA Form 106	Report and complete DEA Form 106

Note: All records must be maintained for 2 years, unless a state requires longer.

* Emergency prescriptions require a signed follow-up prescription. Exceptions: facsimile prescription serves as the original prescription when issued to residents of Long Term Care Facilities, Hospice patients, or compounded IV (i.e. Home Infusion) narcotic medications.

** Where authorized by state controlled substances authority.

What is the DEA Form 224 used for?
Applying for pharmacy DEA registration.

How frequently does a pharmacy's DEA registration need to be renewed?
Every 3 years.

What is the DEA Form 222 used for?
Ordering Schedule I and Schedule II controlled substances.

If you make a mistake when filling out a DEA Form 222 can you just cross out the error?
No, if an error is made then all copies of the 222 form must be voided and retained in your records.

How many carbon copies are attached to a DEA Form 222?
2 copies, so you have the original plus 2 copies.

What color is each copy of a DEA Form 222?
- The first page (original) is brown.
- The second page (first carbon copy) is green.
- The third page (second carbon copy) is blue.

When ordering Schedule II drugs for your pharmacy, what do you do with the first two pages (brown and green) of the DEA Form 222?
Give them to the supplier without separating them. For the form to be valid from the supplier's perspective, the brown and green copies must be intact with the carbon paper between them.

Which part of the DEA Form 222 is the supplier required to retain?
The first page (brown copy).

Which part of the DEA Form 222 does the supplier forward to the DEA?
The second page (green copy).

Which part of the DEA Form 222 is the pharmacy required to retain?
The third page (blue copy).

How long are you required to maintain records of your 222 forms?
2 years.

What is the DEA Form 222a used for?
Ordering more DEA 222 Forms.

What is the DEA Form 106 used for?
Reporting loss or theft of controlled substances.

What is the DEA Form 104 used for?
Closing a pharmacy/surrendering a pharmacy permit.

What is the DEA Form 41 used for?
Reporting the destruction of controlled substances.

BLANK DEA FORM-222
U.S. OFFICIAL ORDER FORM - SCHEDULES I & II

See Reverse of PURCHASER'S Copy of Instructions	No order form may be issued for Schedule I and II substances unless a completed application form has been received, (21 CFR 1305.04).		OMB APPROVAL No. 1117-0010
TO: *(Name of Supplier)*		STREET ADDRESS	
CITY and STATE	DATE	TO BE FILLED IN BY SUPPLIER	
		SUPPLIERS DEA REGISTRATION No.	

LINE No.	No. of Packages	Size of Package	Name of Item	National Drug Code	Packages Shipped	Date Shipped
	TO BE FILLED IN BY PURCHASER					
1						
2						
3						
4						
5						
6						
7						
8						
9						
10						

◀ **LAST LINE COMPLETED** *(MUST BE 10 OR LESS)*   SIGNATURE OR PURCHASER OR ATTORNEY OR AGENT

Date Issued	DEA Registration No.	Name and Address of Registrant
Schedules		
Registered as a	No. of this Order Form	

DEA Form-222
(Oct. 1992)

U.S. OFFICIAL ORDER FORMS - SCHEDULES I & II
DRUG ENFORCEMENT ADMINISTRATION
SUPPLIER'S Copy 1

Note: The graphic illustrated above is only a depiction of the DEA Form-222. It is not intended to be used as an actual order form.

Image from:
http://www.deadiversion.usdoj.gov/pubs/manuals/narcotic/appendixb/222.htm

Doctor of Medicine (MD)
Doctor of Osteopathic Medicine (DO)
Doctor of Dental Medicine (DMD)
Doctor of Dental Surgery (DDS)
Doctor of Optometry (OD)
Doctor of Podiatric Medicine (DPM)
Doctor of Veterinary Medicine (DVM)
Physician Assistant (PA)
Nurse Practitioner (NP)

Can dentists prescribe medications to treat depression?

No, prescribers cannot prescribe medications to treat conditions outside of their scope of practice. For instance, a DVM cannot prescribe medications for a human, a DPM cannot prescribe medications to treat conditions of the eye, an OD cannot prescribe medications to treat conditions of the foot, etc.

Note: In some states, other healthcare professionals may have prescriptive authority (e.g. certified nurse-midwives).

How do I know if a prescriber's DEA number is valid?

There are two components of a DEA number, the letters and the numbers. First we will look at the letters.

The 1ST Letter

DEA numbers begin with 2 letters. The 1st letter of the DEA number provides information about the type of practitioner or registrant.

- A, B, or F for physicians, dentists, veterinarians, hospitals, and pharmacies.
- M for midlevel practitioners.
- P or R for drug distributors.

Note: The DEA number will start with an X for prescribers who have been granted a DEA waiver to write prescriptions for Subutex® or Suboxone® outside of a narcotic treatment program.

The 2ND Letter

The second letter of the DEA number will be the same as the first letter of the prescriber's last name or the first letter in the name of the business.

Now that you know what the letters in a DEA number represent, let's look at the equation to verify a DEA number using the numbers.

Part 1

Add the 2ND, 4TH, and 6TH digits of the DEA number and multiply the sum by 2 to get X.

Note: Remember to multiply the correct set of numbers by 2 (the 2ND, 4TH, and 6TH digits of the DEA number). If you add the 1ST, 3RD, and 5TH digits of the DEA number and multiply that sum by 2, you will get the wrong answer. This is probably the most common mistake people make.

Part 2

Add the 1ST, 3RD, and 5TH digits of the DEA number to get Y.

Part 3

Take your answer from Part 1 and add it to your answer from Part 2 to get Z. In other words, $X + Y = Z$.

Part 4

Your answer from part 3 (Z) will be a 2 digit number. If the DEA number is valid, then the second digit of your two digit answer from Part 3 (Z) will match the 7TH and final digit of the DEA number. For example, let's say your answer from Part 3 was Z = 48. If the DEA number was valid, then the DEA number would end with an 8.

Practice Problem
Verify the example DEA number below.

John Smith, MD
DEA # FS8524616

Solution:
- The registrant is a physician (MD), so the first letter is A, B, or F.
- The prescriber's last name is Smith, so the second letter is S.
- $5 + 4 + 1 = 10$ and $10 \times 2 = 20$... $8 + 2 + 6 = 16$
- The sum of 20 and 16 is 36.
- The last number of the DEA number is 6, which is the same as the last number in the sum of $20 + 16$.
- According to our analysis, this DEA number appears to be valid.

Note: The Drug Addiction Treatment Act of 2000 (DATA 2000) is the name of the law that requires prescribers to include their special DEA number (starting with "X") on prescriptions written for Subutex® or Suboxone®.

How did the Poison Prevention Packaging Act of 1970 change the way we dispense drugs?
This act required drugs to be dispensed in child-resistant packaging (there are several exceptions; one exception is nitroglycerin sublingual tablets).

Why are nitroglycerin sublingual tablets exempt from the PPPA?
Nitroglycerin sublingual tablets are used to restore blood flow to the heart during an exacerbation of angina (characterized by acute chest pain), potentially preventing a myocardial infarction (heart attack). Child resistant packaging may cause an individual on the verge of a heart attack to struggle with opening the container of this potentially life-saving medication (nitroglycerin). As a result, this medication is exempt from the rules of the PPPA.

What is the intent of the PPPA?
The PPPA is intended to protect children from serious injury or illness caused by handling, using, or ingesting medications and certain household substances.

How is this accomplished?
The PPPA protects children by requiring manufacturers to use packaging that is *significantly difficult* for children under the age of 5 years old to open, yet not difficult for normal adults to open.

What is the purpose of the Health Insurance Portability and Accountability Act of 1996 (HIPAA)?
To protect the privacy of individual health information (referred to in the law as "protected health information" or "PHI").

If an individual's PHI has been breached, what must be done according to HIPAA?
The individual must be notified by the person or entity holding the information that their PHI was exposed. This is known as the "HIPAA Breach Notification Rule."

Does HIPAA set standards for protecting *electronic* PHI, such as electronic medical records (EMR)?
Yes.

When using or disclosing PHI, what principle should you keep in mind?
The principle of "minimum necessary use and disclosure."

"Minimum necessary use and disclosure" does not apply to certain situations, which include:
- Disclosures to a healthcare provider for treatment.
- Disclosures to the patient upon request.
- Disclosures authorized by the patient.
- Disclosures necessary to comply with other laws.
- Disclosures to the Dept. of Health and Human Services (HHS) for a compliance investigation, review, or enforcement.

How did the Omnibus Reconciliation Act of 1990 (OBRA '90) change pharmacy practice?
By requiring drug utilization reviews (DUR) and pharmaceutical care (i.e. pharmacist counseling) for Medicaid patients.

If OBRA '90 only requires an offer for pharmacist counseling to be made to Medicaid patients, why does *every* customer (including non-Medicaid customers) receive the same offer?
The "offer to counsel" became part of standard pharmacy business practices to ensure that all customers were receiving the same level of service.

A drug that is compounded cannot be a copy of _____.
A commercially available product.

Manufacturers of bulk products used in compounding must be registered with

_____.
The FDA.

True or false. A pharmacy can advertise compounding of a type of drug (e.g. "We compound bio-identical hormone replacement products").
False, you would need to be registered as a manufacturer to advertise in this manner. A pharmacy cannot promote the compounding of any specific drug, drug class, or type of drug.

What is one of the major issues surrounding bio-identical hormone compounding?
Bio-identical hormone formulations contain estradiol, estrone, estriol, progesterone, and testosterone. Estriol is not an FDA-approved drug, so compounding with estriol is illegal.

Vioxx (rofecoxib) was taken off of the market due to safety concerns. Would it be legal to compound a product containing rofecoxib?
No, the FDA prohibits compounding of drugs that have been deemed unsafe or ineffective.

You compound a drug product without a prescription. Is this okay?
No, this would be considered manufacturing. When compounding, you need to be compounding for a specific prescription.

Pseudoephedrine can only be purchased from what location?
Behind the pharmacy counter or from a locked cabinet stored away from customers.

True or false. Pseudoephedrine can be purchased without a photo ID.
False.

What packaging requirement applies to solid oral dosage forms of pseudoephedrine?
They must be packaged and sold in blister packs, pseudoephedrine can never be sold as loose tablets/capsules.

Daily sales of pseudoephedrine are limited to what amount?
3.6 grams/day.

Monthly (30-day) sales of pseudoephedrine are limited to what amount?
9 grams/30 days.

Federal law limits the amount of pseudoephedrine purchased via mail order to what amount over a 30-day period?
7.5 grams.

What information must be logged during the sale of products containing pseudoephedrine?
- Product name.
- Quantity sold.
- Name and address of purchaser.
- Date and time of sale.
- Signature of purchaser.

Records from pseudoephedrine sales must be kept for what length of time?
2 years.

Restricted Drug Programs

All medications have benefits (the intended therapeutic effect) and risks (side effects). Some drugs have higher risks than others. Those drugs with an unacceptably high level of risk typically do not reach the market or, if they have already reached the market, get withdrawn from the market (e.g. Vioxx®). What do you do when you have a medication with a very high level of risk that has a tremendous benefit for some patients? The answer is - restricted drug programs (also referred to as "REMS"). REMS is an acronym for Risk Evaluation and Mitigation Strategies. The FDA, pursuant to the FDA Amendments Act of 2007, can *require* manufacturers to comply with REMS to manage the risks associated with certain drugs. REMS are meant to ensure that the benefits of using a particular medication outweigh the associated risks.

What consequence can a manufacturer face for failing to comply with REMS?
A fine of at least $250,000 per incident.

Can manufacturers require its own REMS program without being required by the FDA to create such a program?
Yes.

Approximately how many drugs have a REMS program?
Over 100 drugs.

What are some of the most well-known and frequently used REMS programs?
iPLEDGE™, THALIDOMID REMS™., T.I.P.S., and Clozaril® National Registry.

What is iPLEDGE™?
iPLEDGE™ is a REMS program aimed at ensuring patients beginning isotretinoin therapy are not pregnant and preventing pregnancy in patients receiving isotretinoin therapy. Why? When used during pregnancy, isotretinoin has been clearly linked to <u>severe birth defects</u>.

> <u>Note</u>: several brand name formulations of isotretinoin are available: Absorbica®, Accutane®, Amnesteem®, Claravis®, Myorisan®, Sotret®, and Zenatane®.

THALIDOMID REMS™ (formerly known as S.T.E.P.S. ®)
THALIDOMID REMS™ was previously known as S.T.E.P.S.® (System for Thalidomide Education and Prescribing Safety). Thalomid® (thalidomide) can be used for the treatment of multiple myeloma and erythema nodosum leprosum, but the drug causes <u>severe birth defects in unborn babies and venous thromboembolic events (deep vein thrombosis and pulmonary thromboembolism) in patients using the drug</u>. Similar to isotretinoin, thalidomide can never be used in women who are pregnant or may become pregnant.

T.I.P.S.
Tikosyn In Pharmacy System (T.I.P.S.) is a REMS program aimed at communicating the risk of induced arrhythmia with the use of Tikosyn® (dofetilide). Tikosyn® (dofetilide) is used to induce and maintain normal cardiac sinus rhythm in highly symptomatic patients with atrial fibrillation or atrial flutter of more than one week. The major issue with this drug is that it can actually cause potentially fatal ventricular arrhythmias, especially in patients just starting or re-starting therapy. For this reason, patients receiving this drug must be admitted to a facility for close medical monitoring for a minimum of 3 days when starting or re-starting therapy with this drug.

Clozaril® National Registry
The Clozaril® National Registry is essentially a database where the white blood cell count (WBC) for patients receiving therapy with clozapine can be recorded and viewed. Clozaril® (clozapine) is used in the treatment of various psychiatric disorders (e.g. schizophrenia, bipolar disorder). The problem with clozapine is the potentially fatal side effect of agranulocytosis (suppression of white blood cell production). For this reason, white blood cells must be measured by a medical lab and recorded in the Clozaril® National Registry every week for the first 6 months of therapy and periodically thereafter. Pharmacies can only dispense enough of the drug to treat the patient until their next scheduled lab work (e.g. a 7 days' supply every week for the first 6 months of therapy). This program has been referred to as the "no blood, no drug" program.

Do all REMS programs require as much work as iPLEDGE™, THALIDOMID REMS™, T.I.P.S., and the Clozaril® National Registry?
No, in fact some drugs have REMS programs that are so simple you might be surprised they are considered REMS programs at all. One example is Dulera® (mometasone furoate/formoterol). The only requirement for the Dulera® REMS program is that the increased risk of asthma-related death associated with the use of long-acting beta agonists (such as the formoterol found in Dulera®) must be communicated to healthcare professionals and prescribers.

CLINICAL TRIALS

How does a drug get approved by the FDA for use in humans?
Drugs are approved by the FDA after they are proven to be safe and effective. Proof comes from clinical trial data. Clinical trials are comprised of four phases (see below) and the process of obtaining FDA approval usually takes several years.

Phase 1 Clinical Trials
- Small study involving 20 - 80 healthy male volunteers.
- Low doses are tested.
- Collect data on drug bioavailability and dose needed to elicit a response.

Phase 2 Clinical Trials
- Study involving 40 - 300 patients with the disease of interest.
- Minimum effective dose and maximum toxic dose are determined.
- Record side effects experienced by the test subjects.

Phase 3 Clinical Trials
- Study involving 300 – 3,000 patients of various gender, race, lifestyle, and age.
- Assess the risks and benefits of using the drug.
- Refine the drug formulation.
- Conduct placebo studies.

Post-marketing Surveillance
- Continue to gather information about the safety and effectiveness of a drug after it has been approved and marketed.
- Some drugs get removed from the market due to revelations from post-marketing surveillance (e.g. Vioxx® (rofecoxib) was a COX-2 inhibitor removed from the market when post-marketing surveillance revealed an increased risk of cardiovascular events such as heart attack and stroke).

CONTROLLED SUBSTANCE
SCHEDULES

It is important to be able to recognize which schedule a controlled substance belongs to. Below, I have provided you with several practical tips for figuring out which schedule a drug belongs in based on the name of the drug.

Schedule I Controlled Substances

Many Schedule I controlled substances are opiate derivatives. As a result, their names are similar to opiates you have seen used medically. Those used medically fall into Schedule II – V. Below are several example of Schedule I opiates. I have underlined the part of the drug name that should indicate to you that these drugs are opioids.

- Acetyldihydrocodeine ("-codeine" as in codeine)
- Acetylmethadol (-methad- as in methadone)
- Alphacetylmethadol ("-methad-" as in methadone)
- Alphameprodine ("-meprodine" as in meperidine)
- Alphamethadol ("-methad-" as in methadone)
- Alpha-methylfentanyl ("-fentanyl as in fentanyl)
- Betacetylmethadol
- Betameprodine
- Difenoxin ("difenox-" as in diphenoxylate)
- 3-Methylfentanyl
- Morpheridine ("morpheridine" as in morphine and meperidine)
- Norlevorphanol ("-orph-" as in morphine)

Other examples of Schedule I controlled substances are more obvious, such as:

- GHB (Gamma hydroxybutyric acid)
- Heroin
- LSD (Lysergic acid diethylamide)
- Mescaline
- MDMA (3, 4-Methylenedioxymethamphetamine)
- Peyote
- PCP (phencyclidine) analogues
  - Note: phencyclidine (PCP) is C-II

Schedule II Controlled Substances

<u>C-II Opioids:</u>
- Alfentanil — Alfenta
- Alphaprodine
- Anileridine — Leritine
- Bezitramide — Burgodin
- Carfentanil — Wildnil
- Codeine
- Dihydrocodeine
- Dihydroetorphine
- Diphenoxylate
- Ethylmorphine
- Etorphine hydrochloride
- Fentanyl — Fentora, Duragesic, Actiq
- Hydrocodone
- Hydromorphone — Dilaudid
- Isomethadone — Liden
- Levomethorphan
- Levorphanol — Levo-Dromoran
- Metazocine
- Methadone — Dolophine
- Morphine
- Oxycodone — Oxycontin, Roxicodone
- Oxymorphone — Opana
- Pethidine — Demerol
- Phenazocine — Prinadol, Narphen
- Piminodine
- Racemethorphan
- Racemorphan
- Romifentanil
- Sufentanil — Ultiva, Sufenta
- Thebaine

C-II Stimulants:
- Amphetamine
- Cocaine
- Methamphetamine
- Methylphenidate   *Concerta*
- Phenmetrazine
- Phenylacetone

C-II Depressants:
- Amobarbital
- Glutethimide
- Pentobarbital
- Phencyclidine (PCP)
- Phencyclidine (PCP) immediate precursors:
  - 1 -Phenylcyclohexylamine
  - 1 -Piperidinocyclohexanecarbonitrile (PCC)
- Secobarbital   *Seconal*

C-II Hallucinogens:
- Nabilone

                                     Cesamet

Schedule III Controlled Substances

C-III Opioids:
- Paregoric
- Buprenorphine
- Codeine (e.g. Tylenol #3)*
- Dihydrocodeine*
- Dihydrocodeinone*
- Ethylmorphine*
- Morphine*
- Opium*

*In limited quantities <u>in combination with other medications</u>.

C-III Mixed Opioid Agonist/Antagonists:
- Nalorphine

C-III Stimulants:
- Benzphetamine
- Chlorphentermine
- Clortermine
- Phendimetrazine

C-III Depressants:
- Barbituric acid and its derivatives
- Chlorhexadol
- Ketamine
- Lysergic acid
- Lysergic acid amide
  - Note: lysergic acid diethylamide (LSD) is a C-I drug
- Sulfondiethylmethane
- Sulfonethylmethane
- Sulfonmethane
- Tiletamine
- Zolazepam

**These C-II depressants are considered Schedule III when they are used in a compound, mixture, or suppository:
- Amobarbital
- Pentobarbital
- Secobarbital

C-III Anabolic Steroids:

Note: **All anabolic steroids are C-III**

- Boldenone
- Chorionic gonadotropin
- Clostebol
- Dibydrostestosterone
- Drostanolone
- Fluoxymesterone
- Formebulone
- Mesterolene
- Methandienone
- Methandranone
- Methandriol
- Methandrostenolone
- Methenolene
- Methyltestosterone
- Nandrolene
- Nandrolone
- Norethandrolene
- Oxandrolone
- Oxymesterone
- Oxymetholone
- Stanolone
- Stanozolol
- Testolactone
- Testosterone

C-III Hallucinogens:

- Dronabinol

Schedule IV Controlled Substances

C-IV Depressants (Benzodiazepines):
Note: All benzodiazepines are classified as Schedule C-IV. The best way to recognize a benzodiazepine is by the last part of the generic name of the dug. The generic drug name almost always ends in "–pam" or "– lam." Below is a list of benzodiazepines. Exceptions to the naming rule will be pointed out.

- Alprazolam
- Bromazepam
- Camazepam
- Chlordiazepoxide
    - The first benzodiazepine formally discovered
    - The only benzodiazepine that ends in -epoxide.
    - The best way to tell by the name that this is a benzodiazepine is by the -diazep- in the name.
- Clobazam
    - The only benzodiazepine that ends in -zam rather than - lam or -pam.
- Clonazepam
- Clorazepate
    - One of two benzodiazepines that end in -ate.
    - The -aze- is another way to tell by the name that this drug is a benzodiazepine.
- Clotiazepam
- Cloxazolam
- Delorazepam
- Diazepam
- Estazolam
- Ethyl loflazepate
    - Two of two benzodiazepines that end in -ate.
    - Once again, the -aze- is a way to tell by the name that this drug is a benzodiazepine.
- Fludiazepam
- Flunitrazepam
    - Classified as a C-I drug in some states due to the fact that it has been used as a date rape drug.
- Flurazepam
- Halazepam
- Haloxazolam
- Ketazolam

- Loprazolam
- Lorazepam
- Lormetazepam
- Medazepam
- Midazolam
- Nimetazepam
- Nitrazepam
- Nordiazepam
- Oxazepam
- Oxazolam
- Pinazepam
- Prazepam
- Quazepam
- Temazepam
- Tetrazepam
- Triazolam

C-IV Depressants (Other GABA$_A$ Receptor Agonists):
All of these drugs are in Schedule IV, like benzodiazepines they are agonists at GABA$_A$ receptors.

- Eszopiclone
- Zaleplon
- Zolpidem

C-IV Depressants (Sedative-Hypnotics and Anxiolytics):
- Chloral betaine
- Chloral hydrate
- Ethchlorvynol
- Ethinamate
- Mebutamate
- Meprobamate
- Paraldehyde
- Petrichloral

C-IV Depressants (Barbiturates):
- Barbital
  - The first commercially-produced barbiturate
- Methohexital
- Methylphenobarbital (mephobarbital)
- Phenobarbital

C-IV Muscle Relaxants:
- Carisoprodol

C-IV Anti-Obesity Agents:
- Fenfluramine

C-IV Opioids
- Dextro-propoxyphene
    - Also known as propoxyphene
    - Taken off of the market due to an association with potentially fatal cardiac arrhythmias.

Note: tramadol is currently being considered by the DEA for change from non-controlled status to a schedule IV controlled substance.

C-IV Mixed Opioid Agonist/Antagonists:
- Butorphanol
- Pentazocine

C-IV Stimulants:
- Cathine
- Diethylpropion
- Fencamfamin
- Fenproporex
- Mefenorex
- Modafinil
- Muzindol
- Pemoline
- Phentermine
- Sibutramine

Schedule V Controlled Substances

<u>C-V Opioids:</u>
**When the strength per unit dose is very small, these medications are classified as Schedule V.
- Codeine
- Dihydrocodeine
- Diphenoxylate with atropine
  - Lomotil® (diphenoxylate and atropine)
- Ethylmorphine

<u>C-V Stimulants:</u>
- Pyrovalerone

Schedule VI Controlled Substances

There are only two drugs classified as Schedule VI in North Carolina. They are both cannabinoids.

C-VI Cannabinoids:
- Marijuana
- Tetrahydrocannabinols

Congratulations, you are almost prepared to take the North Carolina MPJE®! I would be comfortable taking the exam after studying just the material covered in this book. However, if you have the time and still want more material to review, I would recommend that you also study the following:

- The Frequently Asked Questions (FAQs) on the Board of Pharmacy website (**www.ncbop.org**). The FAQs cover practical topics concerning pharmacy practice in North Carolina. I would try to review as many of these as possible.

- If you really want to know everything, then also consider reading the North Carolina Board of Pharmacy Newsletters. There is a newsletter for each month since 1979 available in a PDF format on the Board of Pharmacy website (**www.ncbop.org**). I would start reading the most recent newsletters and go backward (e.g. 2013, 2012, then 2011... etc) until you get tired of reading them. It is not necessary to read them all.

- You should prioritize your studying as follows:

    1. PHARMACY LAW SIMPLIFIED
    2. Pharmacist FAQs (**www.ncbop.org**)
    3. Board of Pharmacy Newsletters (**www.ncbop.org**)

Do not rush yourself on the exam. Be calm and take your time. One hundred twenty minutes is more than enough time to carefully answer each question on the exam.

Good luck!

NOTES

NOTES

NOTES

NOTES

NOTES